Proximal Biceps

Editor

ANTHONY A. ROMEO

CLINICS IN SPORTS MEDICINE

www.sportsmed.theclinics.com

Consulting Editor
MARK D. MILLER

January 2016 • Volume 35 • Number 1

ELSEVIER

1600 John F. Kennedy Boulevard • Suite 1800 • Philadelphia, Pennsylvania, 19103-2899

http://www.theclinics.com

CLINICS IN SPORTS MEDICINE Volume 35, Number 1
January 2016 ISSN 0278-5919, ISBN-13: 978-0-323-41470-8

Editor: Jennifer Flynn-Briggs
Developmental Editor: Donald Mumford

Clinics in Sports Medicine (ISSN 0278-5919) is published quarterly by Elsevier Inc., 360 Park Avenue South, New York, NY 10010-1710. Months of issue are January, April, July, and October. Business and Editorial Offices: 1600 John F. Kennedy Blvd., Ste. 1800, Philadelphia, PA 19103-2899. Customer Service Office: 3251 Riverport Lane, Maryland Heights, MO 63043. Periodicals postage paid at New York, NY and additional mailing offices. Subscription prices are $340.00 per year (US individuals), $597.00 per year (US institutions), $100.00 per year (US students), $385.00 per year (Canadian individuals), $737.00 per year (Canadian institutions), $235.00 (Canadian students), $470.00 per year (foreign individuals), $737.00 per year (foreign institutions), and $235.00 per year (foreign students). Foreign air speed delivery is included in all *Clinics* subscription prices. All prices are subject to change without notice. **POSTMASTER:** Send address changes to *Clinics in Sports Medicine*, Elsevier Health Sciences Division, Subscription Customer Service, 3251 Riverport Lane, Maryland Heights, MO 63043. Customer Service (orders, claims, online, change of address): Elsevier Health Sciences Division, Subscription Customer Service, 3251 Riverport Lane, Maryland Heights, MO 63043. **Tel: 1-800-654-2452 (U.S. and Canada); 314-447-8871 (outside U.S. and Canada). Fax: 314-447-8029. E-mail: journalscustomerservice-usa@elsevier.com (for print support); journalsonlinesupport-usa@elsevier.com (for online support).**

Reprints. For copies of 100 or more of articles in this publication, please contact the Commercial Reprints Department, Elsevier Inc., 360 Park Avenue South, New York, NY 10010-1710. Tel.: 212-633-3874; Fax: 212-633-3820; E-mail: reprints@elsevier.com.

Clinics in Sports Medicine is covered in *MEDLINE/PubMed (Index Medicus) Current Contents/Clinical Medicine, Excerpta Medica,* and *ISI/Biomed.*

Contributors

CONSULTING EDITOR

MARK D. MILLER, MD
S. Ward Casscells Professor, Head, Division of Sports Medicine, Department of Orthopaedic Surgery, University of Virginia, Charlottesville, Virginia; Team Physician, James Madison University, Harrisonburg, Virginia

EDITOR

ANTHONY A. ROMEO, MD
Professor, Department of Orthopedic Surgery, Section Head, Shoulder and Elbow Surgery, Team Physician, Chicago White Sox and Chicago Bulls, Division of Sports Medicine, Rush University Medical Center, Chicago, Illinois

AUTHORS

KNUT BEITZEL, MA, MD
Orthopaedic Surgeon, Department of Orthopaedic Sports Medicine, Technical University Munich, Munich, Germany

AMRUT BORADE, MD
Division of Shoulder and Elbow Surgery, Department of Orthopaedic Surgery, The Johns Hopkins University, Baltimore, Maryland

JONATHAN BRAVMAN, MD
Associate Professor, Department of Orthopaedics, Sports Medicine and Shoulder Surgery, CU Sports Medicine, University of Colorado Hospital, Boulder, Colorado

STEPHEN F. BROCKMEIER, MD
Associate Professor, Department of Orthopaedic Surgery, University of Virginia, Charlottesville, Virginia

RYAN M. CARR, MD
Shoulder and Elbow Fellow, Cleveland Akron Shoulder and Elbow Fellowship (CASE), Beachwood, Ohio

SIMONE CERCIELLO, MD
Department of Geriatrics, Neurosciences and Orthopaedics, Policlinico Agostino Gemelli, Orthopaedic Surgeon, Catholic University of Rome, Rome, Italy

PETER N. CHALMERS, MD
Orthopaedic Surgery Resident, Department of Orthopaedic Surgery, Rush University Medical Center, Chicago, Illinois

ASHLEY CHRISMAN, PA-C
Physician Assistant, Department of Orthopaedics, CU Sports Medicine, University of Colorado Hospital, Boulder, Colorado

BRIAN J. COLE, MD, MBA
Division of Shoulder and Elbow and Sports Medicine, Department of Orthopaedic Surgery, Rush University Medical Center, Chicago, Illinois

MARK P. COTE, PT, DPT, MSCTR
Sports Medicine Clinical Outcomes Research Facilitator, Department of Orthopaedic Surgery, UConn Musculoskeletal Institute, University of Connecticut, Farmington, Connecticut

REUBEN GOBEZIE, MD
Fellowship Director, Cleveland Akron Shoulder and Elbow Fellowship (CASE); Director, Cleveland Shoulder Institute, University Hospitals of Cleveland, Beachwood, Ohio

PETER HABERMEYER, Prof, MD
Deutsches Schulterzentrum, ATOS Clinic Munich, Munich, Germany

RUSSELL E. HOLZGREFE, BS, BBA
Medical Student, Department of Orthopaedic Surgery, University of Virginia, Charlottesville, Virginia

TODD R. HOOKS, PT, ATC, OCS, SCS, NREMT-1, CSCS, CMTPT, FAAOMPT
New Orleans Pelicans Basketball Team, New Orleans, Louisiana; Myopain Seminars, Bethesda, Maryland

DOMINIC KING, DO
Primary Care Sports Medicine Physician; Associate Staff Physician, Cleveland Clinic Center for Sports Health, Garfield Heights, Ohio

FRANK MARTETSCHLÄGER, MD, PhD
Deutsches Schulterzentrum, ATOS Clinic Munich; Department of Orthopaedic Sports Medicine, Klinikum rechts der Isar, Technical University Munich, Munich, Germany

AUGUSTUS D. MAZZOCCA, MS, MD
Professor and Chairman, Department of Orthopaedic Surgery; Director, UConn Musculoskeletal Institute, UConn Health, Director of Clinical Biomechanics and the Bioskills Laboratory, University of Connecticut, Farmington, Connecticut

ERIC McCARTY, MD
Chief of Sports Medicine and Shoulder Surgery, Associate Professor, Department of Orthopaedics, CU Sports Medicine, University of Colorado Hospital, Boulder, Colorado

EDWARD G. McFARLAND, MD
Division of Shoulder and Elbow Surgery, Department of Orthopaedic Surgery, The Johns Hopkins University, Baltimore, Maryland

GREGORY P. NICHOLSON, MD
Associate Professor, Division of Shoulder and Elbow and Sports Medicine, Department of Orthopaedic Surgery, Rush University Medical Center, Chicago, Illinois

STEPHEN J. O'BRIEN, MD, MBA
Clinical Professor of Orthopaedic Surgery, Weill Cornell Medical College; Attending Surgeon, Department of Sports Medicine and Shoulder Surgery, Hospital for Special Surgery, New York, New York

KUSHAL V. PATEL, MD
Baylor Scott and White Orthopaedics at Garland, Garland, Texas

MARK SCHICKENDANTZ, MD
Orthopaedic Surgeon; Director, Cleveland Clinic Center for Sports Health; Associate Professor of Surgery, Cleveland Clinic Lerner College of Medicine, Garfield Heights, Ohio

YOUSEF SHISHANI, MD
Research Fellow, Cleveland Shoulder Institute, University Hospitals of Cleveland, Beachwood, Ohio

MARK TAUBER, MD, PhD
Deutsches Schulterzentrum, ATOS Clinic Munich, Munich, Germany; Department of Traumatology and Sports Injuries, Paracelsus Medical University, Salzburg, Austria

SAMUEL A. TAYLOR, MD
Assistant Professor of Orthopaedic Surgery, Weill Cornell Medical College; Assistant Attending Surgeon, Department of Sports Medicine and Shoulder Surgery, Hospital for Special Surgery, New York, New York

NIKHIL N. VERMA, MD
Associate Professor, Department of Orthopaedic Surgery, Rush University Medical Center, Chicago, Illinois

ARMANDO VIDAL, MD
Associate Professor, Department of Orthopaedics, Sports Medicine and Shoulder Surgery, CU Sports Medicine, University of Colorado Hospital, Boulder, Colorado

MANDEEP S. VIRK, MD
Divisions of Shoulder and Elbow and Sports Medicine, Department of Orthopaedic Surgery, Rush University Medical Center, Chicago, Illinois; Division of Shoulder and Elbow Surgery, Department of Orthopaedic Surgery, NYU-Langone Medical Center, NYU-Hospital for Joint Diseases, New York, New York

ANDREAS VOSS, MD
Sports Medicine Research Fellow, Department of Orthopaedic Surgery, UConn Musculoskeletal Institute, University of Connecticut, Farmington, Connecticut

BRIAN C. WERNER, MD
Clinical Fellow, Department of Sports Medicine and Shoulder Surgery, Hospital for Special Surgery, New York, New York

KEVIN E. WILK, PT, DPT, FAPTA
Champion Sports Medicine, A Physiotherapy Associates Clinic, Birmingham, Alabama; Rehabilitation Consultant, Tampa Bay Rays Baseball Team, Tampa Bay, Florida; Adjunct Assistant Professor, Physical Therapy Programs, Marquette University, Milwaukee, Wisconsin

JUSTIN YANG, MD
Sports Medicine Fellow, Department of Orthopaedic Surgery, UConn Musculoskeletal Institute, University of Connecticut, Farmington, Connecticut

Contents

 Video of an arthroscopic active compression test with arthroscope in the posterior viewing portal demonstrating incarceration of the long head of the biceps tendon between humeral head and glenoid accompanies this article

The biceps-labral complex represents the shared anatomic and clinical features of the biceps and labrum. It has 3 clinically relevant zones: inside, the superior labrum and the biceps anchor; junction, the intra-articular portion of the long head of the biceps tendon and its stabilizing pulley; and bicipital tunnel, the extra-articular long head of the biceps tendon from the articular margin through the subpectoral region and its fibro-osseous confinement. By embracing this more comprehensive understanding of the anatomy, pathoanatomy, and functional implications, clinicians can proceed with greater confidence and can more accurately select patient-specific surgical techniques.

The biceps reflection pulley is a soft tissue sling that stabilizes the long head of the biceps tendon (LHB) before it enters the bicipital groove. Injuries to the biceps pulley and related instability of the LHB are common diagnoses in patients with anterior shoulder pain. This article summarizes the current concepts for treatment of injuries to the biceps pulley. Clinical and radiological presentation, arthroscopic assessment, and current treatment options are outlined.

The examination of the shoulder for conditions involving the biceps tendon continues to be challenging. Numerous examination tests for biceps and superior labrum anterior and posterior (SLAP) lesions have been scientifically evaluated. This section reports on how to perform these tests and summarizes the clinical utility of the tests. Many of the tests for the examination of the biceps and for SLAP lesions do not have high sensitivity and specificity, which limits their usefulness. Although the dynamic shear test has promise for making the diagnosis of SLAP lesions, the studies reporting its clinical utility are disparate.

Biceps tendon pain is frequently called biceps "tendinitis," or inflammation of the biceps tendon. Histologic analysis of biceps tendon biopsies demonstrates changes in tenocyte size, ground substance, collagen organization, and vascularity observed with many different tendinopathies. There are distinct symptoms of biceps tendinopathy and a few provocative maneuvers can help make the diagnosis. Imaging studies (eg, MRI) can show changes in signal sequence or tears. However, MRI has a low sensitivity and frequently results in missed or misdiagnosed biceps pathology. Clinical decision making is best guided by a strong clinical suspicion based on patient history, physical examination, and MRI.

Nonoperative management of conditions of the long head of biceps tendon (LHBT) involves a multifaceted approach, addressing the entire shoulder complex in addition to conditions that involve the LHBT. LHBT pathologic conditions are divided into 3 categories: inflammation, instability and rupture. This article provides an overview of a nonoperative treatment algorithm that addresses these specific categories and includes a review of ultrasound-guided injection techniques used in the diagnosis and management of LHBT disorders.

The long head of the biceps has garnered increased attention and interest due to the high prevalence of pain that can be a primary condition or occur secondary to shoulder dysfunction. The successful treatment of biceps tendinopathy is dependent on an accurate diagnosis and recognizing all causative factors. The treatment program will be individualized with a rehabilitation program designed to restore strength and flexibility and restore normal tendon mechanics.

Long head biceps tendon is a common cause of anterior shoulder pain. Failure of conservative treatment may warrant surgical intervention. Surgical treatment involves long head biceps tenotomy or tenodesis. Several different techniques have been described for biceps tenodesis, including arthroscopic versus open and suprapectoral versus subpectoral. Most studies comparing tenodesis to tenotomy are limited by the level of evidence and confounding factors, such as concomitant rotator cuff tear.

Many studies demonstrate similar outcomes for both procedures. Surgeon preference is likely more influential in choosing between tenotomy and tenodesis. Higher-powered studies are necessary to elucidate any differences in outcomes if present.

Current arthroscopic surgical techniques for the management of proximal biceps tendon disorders encompass 3 commonly advocated procedures: proximal biceps anchor reattachment (superior labrum anterior to posterior or SLAP repair), biceps tenotomy, and arthroscopic biceps tenodesis. The indications for each procedure vary based on injury pattern, symptomatic presentation, concomitant pathologic abnormality, and most notably, patient factors, such as age, functional demand, and specific sport or activity participation. Outcomes after SLAP repair are generally favorable, although recent studies have found biceps tenodesis to be the preferred treatment for certain patient populations.

This article summarizes both the various techniques for an open subpectoral biceps tenodesis as well as the biomechanics associated with these procedures. It provides information regarding the indications and contraindications to support the surgeon's decision. Furthermore, a postoperative protocol as well as an outcome overview is presented to address postoperative care. A short summary of the recent literature regarding potential complications is included to provide further insight on this technique. The open subpectoral tenodesis of the long head of the biceps is a safe and reproducible technique with a low complication rate for patients with pathologies of the proximal biceps.

The long head of biceps tendon (LHBT) is frequently involved in rotator cuff tears and can cause anterior shoulder pain. Tendon hypertrophy, hourglass contracture, delamination, tears, and tendon instability in the bicipital groove are common macroscopic pathologic findings affecting the LHBT in the presence of rotator cuff tears. Failure to address LHBT disorders in the setting of rotator cuff tear can result in persistent shoulder pain and poor satisfaction after rotator cuff repair. Tenotomy or tenodesis of the LHBT are effective options for relieving pain arising from the LHBT in the setting of reparable and selected irreparable rotator cuff tears.

The proximal long head of the biceps tendon and its attachment at the superior glenoid tubercle and labrum are subject to a spectrum of disorders in overhead athletes. Biceps disorders are commonly characterized by intermittent anterior or deep-seated shoulder pain exacerbated by activity. Diagnosis is reached via various physical examination maneuvers; MRI can be uncertain. Nonsteroidal anti-inflammatory medications, targeted ultrasound-guided corticosteroid injections, and supervised physical therapy are the mainstays of nonoperative treatment. Operative treatment, which remains controversial, provides reliable pain relief, restoration of function for activities of daily living, and low complication rates, but return to play can be unpredictable.

The long head of biceps tendon (LHBT) is a well-recognized cause of anterior shoulder pain. Tenotomy or tenodesis of the LHBT is an effective surgical solution for relieving pain arising from the LHBT. Cosmetic deformity of the arm, cramping or soreness in the biceps muscle, and strength deficits in elbow flexion and supination are the three most common adverse events associated with tenotomy of the LHBT. Complications associated with tenodesis of the LHBT include loss of fixation resulting in cosmetic deformity, residual groove pain, pain or soreness in the biceps muscle, infection, stiffness, hematoma, neurologic injury, vascular injury, proximal humerus fracture, and reflex sympathetic dystrophy.

CLINICS IN SPORTS MEDICINE

RELATED INTEREST

Radiologic Clinics of North America, July 2015 (Vol. 53, Issue 4)
Emergency and Trauma Radiology
Savvas Nicolaou, *Editor*
Available at: http://www.radiologic.theclinics.com/

THE CLINICS ARE AVAILABLE ONLINE!
Access your subscription at:
www.theclinics.com

Foreword

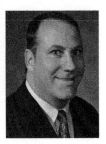

Mark D. Miller, MD
Consulting Editor

I would be hard pressed to name any condition in sports medicine that has received as much attention as proximal biceps injuries has in the last several years. Ten years ago, I rarely, if ever, performed a biceps tenodesis. Today, it is one of the most common procedures that I do. I suspect that we now recognize these injuries more frequently than we did in the past (we didn't see it, but it saw us); however, one could argue that we are now overtreating these injuries. Like everything in our profession, the pendulum swings.

Dr Tony Romeo, a recognized expert in this area, has done an outstanding job in covering this controversial topic. The anatomy, biomechanics, diagnosis, and treatment of proximal biceps tendon injuries are covered in detail in this treatise. All aspects of treatment (nonoperative vs operative management, tenotomy vs tenodesis, arthroscopic vs open tenodesis) are covered in detail. Although the controversy will likely continue, I think we can all learn something from this issue. Thank-you to Dr Romeo and all the authors who contributed to this issue of *Clinics in Sports Medicine*.

Mark D. Miller, MD
University of Virginia
James Madison University
400 Ray C. Hunt Drive, Suite 330
Charlottesville, VA 22908-0159, USA

E-mail address:
MDM3P@hscmail.mcc.virginia.edu

Clin Sports Med 35 (2016) xiii
http://dx.doi.org/10.1016/j.csm.2015.10.012
0278-5919/16/$ – see front matter © 2016 Published by Elsevier Inc.

Preface

The Proximal Biceps Tendon

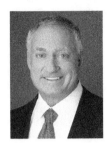

Anthony A. Romeo, MD
Editor

The long head of the biceps has been the subject of much debate in sports medicine. Some surgeons are convinced that it plays an important role in the proprioception and stability of the shoulder, while others suggest it is nothing more than a vestigial structure that can be removed from the glenohumeral joint without consequence. Most surgeons will agree that the tendon and its surrounding structures can be a source of significant pain that may interfere with the function of the shoulder. But understanding the pathology, the reason for pain and dysfunction, and the tendon interaction with other structures such as the superior labrum and rotator cuff is complex and enigmatic. As we continue to evolve our knowledge of this structure, we often find more questions than answers, but more frequently, the answer is to remove the structure from the glenohumeral joint.

This issue is a comprehensive guide to the evaluation and management, both nonsurgical and surgical, of the long head of the biceps tendon. It begins with a discussion of its complex anatomy and biomechanics and then progresses through the physical examination and imaging modalities used to identify its pathologic conditions. A thorough discussion regarding the nonsurgical management and surgical management then ensues, focusing on methods of proximal anchor repair (SLAP repair), to biceps tenotomy and tenodesis. Furthermore, one cannot review the biceps without including a discussion of the subsets of patients that often present with pathology to the long head of the biceps tendon: patients with rotator cuff disease and overhead athletes.

I am indebted to the authors, who are all renowned clinicians and surgeons with a passionate interest in understanding and treating the complexities of the proximal biceps tendon. Each article is a succinct effort to provide a clear understanding of the subject matter and is filled with insights that clearly represent the desire to educate and augment our understanding of the current nonoperative and operative

Clin Sports Med 35 (2016) xv–xvi
http://dx.doi.org/10.1016/j.csm.2015.10.011
0278-5919/16/$ – see front matter © 2016 Published by Elsevier Inc.

sportsmed.theclinics.com

management of the long head of the biceps. Their efforts have created a fantastic resource to guide challenging decisions related to the long head of the biceps tendon.

Anthony A. Romeo, MD
Department of Orthopedic Surgery
Shoulder and Elbow Surgery
Division of Sports Medicine
Rush University Medical Center
1611 West Harrison, Suite 300
Chicago, IL 60612, USA

E-mail address:
anthony.romeo@rushortho.com
Website: http://www.shoulderelbowsports.com

Clinically Relevant Anatomy and Biomechanics of the Proximal Biceps

Samuel A. Taylor, MD*, Stephen J. O'Brien, MD, MBA

KEYWORDS

• Biceps-labral complex • Proximal biceps • Bicipital tunnel

KEY POINTS

• The biceps-labral complex (BLC) represents the shared anatomic and clinical features of the biceps and labrum.
• The BLC has 3 clinically relevant zones: inside, junction, and bicipital tunnel.
• Embracing this more comprehensive understanding of the anatomy, pathoanatomy, and functional implications, clinicians can proceed with greater confidence and more accurately select patient-specific surgical techniques.

Video of an arthroscopic active compression test with arthroscope in the posterior viewing portal demonstrating incarceration of the long head of the biceps tendon between humeral head and glenoid accompanies this article at http://www.sportsmed.theclinics.com/

INTRODUCTION

The long head of the biceps tendon (LHBT) and the glenoid labrum have long been recognized as separate entities. This common misconception has been challenged by recent clinical and basic science efforts. Interpretation of the clinically relevant anatomy, pathoanatomy, and biomechanics of the proximal biceps, therefore, demands a more comprehensive understanding of the glenoid labrum, the intra-articular LHBT, its stabilizing pulley, and the bicipital tunnel. As such, the authors prefer the term biceps-labral complex (BLC) to describe relevant anatomy as it relates to the proximal biceps. To consider one without the others may lead to inaccurate diagnosis and inappropriate selection of surgical technique.

Department of Sports Medicine and Shoulder Surgery, Hospital for Special Surgery, New York, NY, USA
* Corresponding author.
E-mail address: taylors@HSS.edu

Clin Sports Med 35 (2016) 1–18
http://dx.doi.org/10.1016/j.csm.2015.08.005
0278-5919/16/$ – see front matter © 2016 Elsevier Inc. All rights reserved.
sportsmed.theclinics.com

The BLC has 3 clinically relevant zones: inside, junction, and tunnel.[1] Inside includes the superior labrum and the biceps anchor. Junction includes the intra-articular portion of the LHBT and its stabilizing pulley, which is visualized during standard glenohumeral arthroscopy. Bicipital tunnel represents the extra-articular LHBT from the articular margin through the subpectoral region and its fibro-osseous confinement termed the bicipital tunnel (**Fig. 1**).[1,2]

ANATOMY AND FUNCTION
Inside

Glenoid labrum

- The glenoid is a triangular collagenous structure[3] 4 to 6 mm wide and 4 mm thick[4] that is circumferentially connected to the glenoid and acts to deepen the shallow fossa without altering its radius of curvature. It is intimately associated with capsular ligaments.[5]
- Variations of normal anterior labral anatomy (sublabral foramen and Buford complex) must be differentiated from pathologic lesions at arthroscopy.[3,6–9]

Superior labrum

- Morphologic heterogeneity with regard to its attachment to the superior glenoid: In their classic evaluation of 42 shoulder specimens, Cooper and colleagues[3] reported that the morphology of the superior labrum was distinct from the inferior

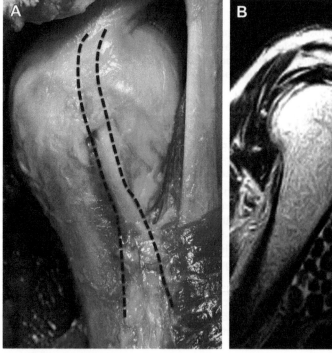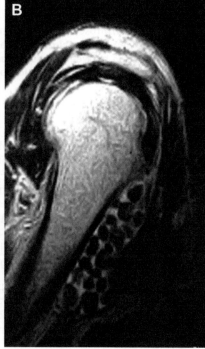

Fig. 1. (*A*) The bicipital tunnel is a closed space (*dashed line*) that extends from the articular margin through the subpectoral region where space-occupying lesions such as loose bodies (*B*) can aggregate and become symptomatic.

labrum. They identified a meniscal loose attachment consisting of thin elastic connective tissue as opposed to a firm inelastic attachment noted for the inferior labrum.

- The posterosuperior labrum closely resembles the LHBT with regard to its collagen component, whereas the anterosuperior labrum contains more elastic fibers and semicircular fibers.[10] Tuoheti and colleagues[11] described an all posterior or posterior-dominated histologic origin of the LHBT from the labrum in 83.1% of 101 cadaveric specimens examined.[12] The elasticity of the anterosuperior labrum, particularly in a zone that connects the glenohumeral ligament to the biceps tendon, may be needed to accept tensile stress within the rotator interval in this region.[13]
- There is a normally occurring synovial reflection at the superior aspect of the glenoid deep to the superior labrum, which is of variable depth. Meniscoid superior labrum is represented by redundant labrum with a deep synovial reflection without tearing of its attachment. Rispoli and colleagues[14] identified 2.6 mm to 7.3 mm overlap of the labrum onto the bony surface of the glenoid. This is a variation of normal anatomy and should not be mistaken for a superior labrum anterior to posterior (SLAP) tear. A mobile and loosely attached superior labrum should not be considered abnormal unless there is definitive detachment and visualized tear.[15]
- Vascularity of the glenoid labrum is based on an anastomotic network from suprascapular, anterior humeral circumflex, and the posterior humeral circumflex artery contributions.[3] Circumferential and radial branches occur without any direct vascularity emanating from the glenoid bone. The most vascularly deprived region of labrum is superior and anterior, which may result in decreased healing potential at these zones.

Biceps anchor

- The LHBT anchor is intimately associated with the superior glenoid labrum[3] in addition to a direct attachment to the supraglenoid tubercle at the 12 o'clock position approximately 5 mm medial to the superior edge of the glenoid rim.
- In a cadaveric study of 105 specimens, Vangsness and colleagues[16] demonstrated that the LHBT attached from the supraglenoid tubercle in 50% of specimens and from the superior labrum in the remaining 50% of specimens. They described 4 types of biceps attachments to the glenoid labrum:
  - Type I attaches to entirely to the posterior labrum
  - Type II is predominately posterior with some anterior labral attachment
  - Type III attaches equally to the anterior and posterior labrum
  - Type IV is mostly anterior labral contribution.

Most biceps tendons that originate from the superior labrum do so posteriorly to the supraglenoid tubercle, a type I or type II labrum.[16,17] The fibers of the LHBT and glenoid labrum blend in this region[3] regardless of their gross appearance.[12] More recently, another large cadaveric study found that 83% of LHBT origins were posterior entirely (28%) or posterior-dominant (55%).[12] A review of 3000 arthroscopic cases showed that there was significant variation with regard to the intra-articular portion of the LHBT ranging from mesotendon, that is freely movable and unattached to the rotator cuff, to an adherent type LHBT in which the LHBT is attached to the supraspinatus and/or labrum.[18] Congenital absence,[19] extra-articular origin,[20] and other variations[21] of the LHBT have also been described.

Junction

Intra-articular long head of the biceps tendon

- The average length of the LHBT from its origin at the supraglenoid tubercle to the musculotendinous junction is 99 to 138 mm.[1,22,23] The average diameter of the LHBT is 6.6 mm for its intra-articular segment and 5.1 to 6 mm for the extra-articular segment.[22,24] In their series of over 200 subjects, Braun and colleagues[25] determined the average diameter of the LHBT at arthroscopy was 6 mm.
- The LHBT requires 19 mm of excursion to take the shoulder through a normal range of motion in the scapular plane.[26]
- The blood supply to the LHBT comes from superior labrum tributaries proximally[3] and ascending branches of the anterior humeral circumflex artery distally. This creates a hypovascular, watershed region 12 to 30 mm from the LHBT origin, corresponding with the segment of tendon that crosses the articular margin, which is a region of the tendon particularly susceptible to rupture.[27]
- The LHBT has neural elements associated with nociception. Alpantaki and colleagues[28] demonstrated an extensive sensory and sympathetic network within the LHBT, densest within the proximal segment of tendon. A follow-up study identified neural cell adhesion molecules that play an important role in nociception within several samples of LHBT harvested from 6 subjects who underwent shoulder surgery.[29] Tosounidis and colleagues[30] used immunohistochemical analysis and identified increased sympathetic innervation of the LHBT with alpha-1 adrenergic receptors identified among subjects with acute proximal humerus fracture and chronic rotator cuff disease compared with cadaveric controls.
- Intra-articular delivery of the LHBT during glenohumeral arthroscopy with a probe is considered the gold standard diagnostic modality for the discovery of pathologic lesions.[31] Hart and colleagues[32] determined that positioning the arm in 30° forward flexion, 40° abduction, and 90° elbow flexion maximized visualization of the LHBT during standard diagnostic arthroscopy.

Biceps pulley

- The biceps pulley is a capsuloligamentous complex that stabilizes the LHBT within the proximal portion of the groove (zone 1 of the bicipital tunnel). The biceps pulley is formed by a coalescence of fibers from the superior glenohumeral ligament, the coracohumeral ligament (CHL), and contributions from the subscapularis and supraspinatus tendons. Together these structures stabilize the LHBT as it turns 35° to 40° along the articular margin en route to its extra-articular position.[33]
- The CHL, often appearing as 2 bands stretching from the coracoid process to the greater tuberosity and partially to the lesser tuberosity, is an inferior stabilizer of the glenohumeral joint. The superior glenohumeral ligament originates with or just anterior to the origin of the LHBT. It consists of oblique and direct fibers that arise from the supraglenoid tubercle and labrum, respectively, parallel with the biceps tendon and inserts onto the fovea capitis just superior to the lesser tuberosity. Some fibers continue to insert into the base of the bicipital groove; the remainder contribute to the transverse humeral ligament.[13,34,35]
- Braun and colleagues[25] defined the arthroscopic anatomy of the biceps pulley as having an anteromedial biceps reflection pulley and a posterolateral biceps

reflection pulley, either of which may become compromised. In their series of 207 subjects who underwent shoulder arthroscopy for a wide variety of pathologic conditions, they found that 32% of subjects had a pulley tear that was highly associated with proximal LHBT instability. Interestingly, there was only a slightly higher predominance of anteromedial pulley lesions than posteromedial. The average age of subjects with pulley tears was 13 years older than those without and there was a significant association of pulley lesions with rotator cuff tears and SLAP tears.

- Biceps excursion at the level of the biceps pulley is 10 to 13 mm with the highest shear forces occurring with the arm in internal rotation with the arm at the side and forward flexion with the humerus in either internal or neutral rotation.[36] These cadaveric finding suggested a vulnerability of the biceps pulley to injury due to increased shear stresses incurred in the aforementioned positions as well as attritional abrasion secondary to repeated excursion of the LHBT against the pulley.

Bicipital Tunnel

Several groups have begun to evaluate the extra-articular segment of the LHBT[2,22,32,37,38] and its clinical implications.[1,39,40] Recently, Taylor and colleagues[2] defined the bicipital tunnel as the fibro-osseous enclosure of the extra-articular LHBT extending from the articular margin through the subpectoral region that often conceals hidden lesions **(Fig. 2)**.[1]

Bicipital tunnel

- Zone 1 represents the traditional bony groove beginning at the articular margin (biceps pulley) and extending to the distal margin of the subscapularis **(Fig. 3)**.[2]
  - Bicipital groove osteology has been implicated in pathogenesis of biceps disease. A prospective study comparing subjects with chronic BLC symptoms (n = 37) versus a group of negative controls (n = 30) using ultrasound and radiographs found a high degree of variation of the depth, width, and contour of the osseous groove.[41] Furthermore, nearly half (44%) of subjects with sonographic evidence of biceps disease also had degenerative changes of the bicipital groove. Cone and colleagues[42] performed a comprehensive evaluation of the osseous groove architecture. Although significant individual variation existed among specimens, they reported the average medial wall angle to be 56°, depth 4.3 mm, top width 8.8 mm, and middle width 5.4 mm. More than 33% of specimens had osteophytes on either the medial wall or floor of the groove.
  - The transverse humeral ligament provides constraint to the LHBT proximally in zone 1. However, in a cadaveric study using MRI and histology, Gleason and colleagues[43] showed that the transverse humeral ligament was, in fact, a continuation of the superficial fibers of the subscapularis tendon stretching over the intertubercular groove that meshed with longitudinal fibers from the supraspinatus and the CHL. Another study[44] reported similar findings in a large cadaveric study of 85 specimens. Specifically, the investigators did not identify a discernable transverse humeral ligament in any specimen. Rather, superficial subscapularis fibers formed this structure in 86% of specimens. Interestingly, 33% of specimens also had subscapularis fibers extending deep to the LHBT along the floor of the groove.
  - In their histologic evaluation, Taylor and colleagues[2] noted that the floor of zone 1 was defined by a deep osseous morphology and a continuation of

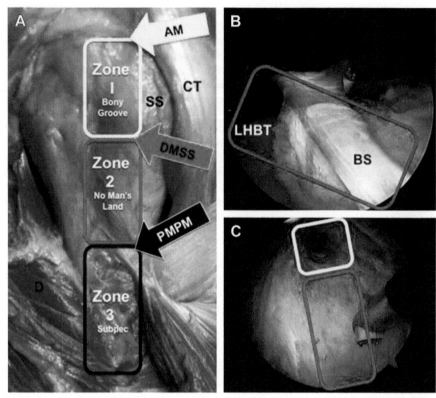

Fig. 2. A soft tissue sheath (*A, B*) consistently covers the LHBT to the level of the proximal margin of the pectoralis major tendon (PMPM) and contributes to the roof of the bicipital tunnel. The sheath is clearly visible during open procedures (*A*) and extra-articular arthroscopic procedures within the subdeltoid space (*B, C*). The fibro-osseous bicipital tunnel consists of 3 distinct anatomic zones (*A*). Zone 1 represents the traditional bony bicipital groove (*yellow box*) beginning at the articular margin (AM) and ending at the distal margin of the subscapularis tendon (DMSS). Zone 2 (*red box*) extends from the DMSS to the PMPM and represents a "no man's land" because it is not viewable from arthroscopy above or from subpectoral exposure below. Zone 3 is distal to the PMPM and represents the subpectoral (Subpec) region. The sheath overlying zone 2 can be robust (*B*). BS, bicipital sheath; CT, conjoint tendon; D, deltoid; SS, subscapularis. (*From* Taylor SA, Fabricant PD, Bansal M, et al. The anatomy and histology of the bicipital tunnel of the shoulder. J Shoulder Elbow Surg 2015;24(4):513; with permission.)

subscapularis tendon fibers and periosteum. Synovium was present in all specimens in zone 1. The roof was composed of blending fibers from the subscapularis and supraspinatus as well as perpendicularly oriented (parallel to LHBT) fibers of the falciform ligament in a subset (33%) of specimens.

- Zone 2 ("no man's land") is the region between the distal margin of the subscapularis and the proximal margin of the pectoralis major tendon and gets its name because this region cannot be visualized by arthroscopy above or from open subpectoral exposure below (see **Fig. 3**).
  - The osseous floor is a shallow trough covered by intersecting fibers of the latissimus dorsi and subscapularis and periosteum. The roof consisted of a circumferential biceps sheath consisting of axially oriented dense connective

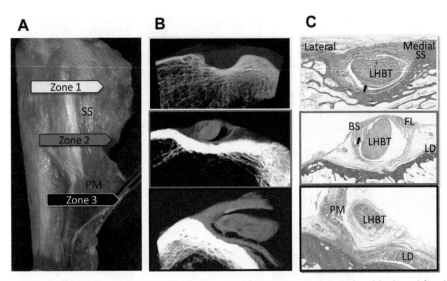

Fig. 3. Using a cadaveric model, the entire bicipital tunnel was harvested en block and fixed in formalin (*A*). Cross-sections were then taken from each of the 3 zones of the bicipital tunnel including zone 1 (*yellow*), zone 2 (*red*), and zone 3 (*black*) (PM, pectoralis major tendon; SS, Subscapularis). Plain radiographs were taken (*B*) demonstrating the osseous architecture of the bicipital tunnel floor from each zone. Histologic evaluation (*C*) demonstrated that zones 1 and 2 were consistently enclosed by dense connective tissue and contained synovium. Zone 3 had significantly more percent empty tunnel and lacked the same dense connective tissue boundaries. Zone 1 (*top right*) shows continuation of the SS fibers superficial and deep to the long head of the biceps tendon (LHBT), which blend with fibers of the supraspinatus laterally. Synovium (*arrow*) completely envelops the LHBT. Zone 2 (*middle right*) demonstrates the axially oriented circumferential fiber of the bicipital sheath (BS), which extended laterally to bone. The falciform ligament (FL) can be seen as a discrete superficial bundle of longitudinally oriented fibers along the medial aspect of the bicipital tunnel. Partial synovial extension is seen (*arrow*). Proximal extension of latissimus dorsi (LD) fibers is also seen in a subset of specimens. Zone 3 (*bottom right*) shows thick fibers of the LD along the floor with a roof of PM. Medially, loose areolar connective tissue predominated. (*From* Taylor SA, Fabricant PD, Bansal M, et al. The anatomy and histology of the bicipital tunnel of the shoulder. J Shoulder Elbow Surg 2015;24(4):511–9.)

tissue fibers and perpendicularly oriented fibers of the falciform ligament.[2] The finding that the falciform ligament and bicipital sheath are separate entities exists in contrast to some previous reports.[45–47] The falciform ligament (**Fig. 4**) is an expansion of the sternocostal head of the pectoralis major but has substantial variability with regard to the location of fibers, its proximal extension, and thickness. Histologic evaluation clearly demonstrated that the falciform ligament had predominantly longitudinally oriented fibers that were superficial to and distinct from the axially oriented fibers of the bicipital sheath. The thickness of these 2 structures was variable among specimens. A minority of specimens (33%) demonstrated continuation of fibers from the falciform ligament into zone 1. Furthermore, only 33% of specimens proved to have a broad investing proximal expansion along the bicipital tunnel as previously reported.[45–47]

○ It is important to note that, despite traditional teaching,[46] there is a synovial reflection in the groove (zone 1); 67% of specimens had synovial tissue identified in zone 2.

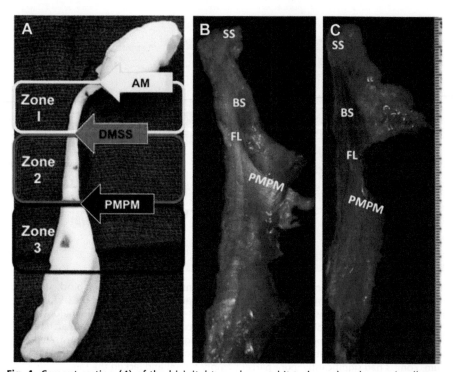

Fig. 4. Cement casting (*A*) of the bicipital tunnel proved it to be a closed space in all specimens. After cement casting, the soft tissue roof of the bicipital tunnel was resected (*B, C*). Whereas the quality of this constraining soft tissue was highly variable among specimens, ranging from robust (*B*) to gossamer (*C*), it was structurally competent and contained the cement in all specimens. AM, articular margin; BS, bicipital sheath; DMSS, distal margin of subscapularis tendon; FL, falciform ligament; PMPM, proximal margin of pectoralis major tendon; SS, subscapularis. (*From* Taylor SA, Fabricant PD, Bansal M, et al. The anatomy and histology of the bicipital tunnel of the shoulder. J Shoulder Elbow Surg 2015;24(4):515; with permission.)

- Zone 3 is a subpectoralis region that extends distal to the proximal margin of the pectoralis major tendon.[2]
  - The floor of this zone is characterized by a flat osseous architecture covered by latissimus dorsi tendon fibers and periosteum.
  - In contrast to zones 1 and 2, the medial enclosure of the LHBT consisted of loose connective tissue for most specimens.
  - Partial extension of synovium was identified in 18% of specimens.
  - The bicipital tunnel was consistently demonstrated to be a closed space. In fact, the percent empty tunnel (%ET) determined by cross-sectional quantitative analysis was similar for zones 1 and 2. Zone 3, however, offered significantly more %ET than either zone 1 or zone 2.

Other Considerations

Limitations of diagnostic arthroscopy

- The average LHBT excursion afforded by arthroscopic pull-test was 15 to 19 mm in cadaveric studies[1,37] and 14 mm in vivo.[38]

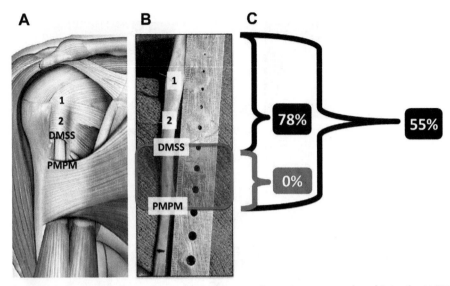

Fig. 5. Using a cadaveric model, percutaneous tagging sutures were placed into the LHBT with the tendon at rest (*A1, B1*) and after maximum tendon excursion applied by arthroscopic grasper (*A2, B2*). The specimens were dissected and the distal margin of the subscapularis (DMSS) and the proximal margin of the pectoralis major (PMPM) were marked on the LHBT and used to calculate the percentage of tendon that can be visualized during glenohumeral arthroscopy (*C*), which was 78% relative to the DMSS and 55% relative to the PMPM.[1] Zone 2 of the bicipital tunnel was named "no man's land" because it cannot be visualized from above or below. (*Adapted from* Taylor SA, Khair MM, Gulotta LV, et al. Diagnostic glenohumeral arthroscopy fails to fully evaluate the biceps-labral complex. Arthroscopy 2015;31(2):215–24; with permission.)

- Hart and colleagues[32] showed that position of the arm in 30° of forward flexion, 40° of abduction, and 90° of elbow flexion maximizes LHBT excursion during diagnostic arthroscopy and the pull-test.
- Using a cadaver model (**Fig. 5**), Taylor and colleagues[1] demonstrated that standard diagnostic arthroscopy using the pull-test, was only able to visualize 78% and 55% of the LHBT relative to the inferior margin of the subscapularis tendon (zone 1) and the proximal margin of the pectoralis major tendon (zone 2), respectively. In a clinical study, Gilmer and colleagues[38] determined that diagnostic arthroscopy with inclusion of the pull-test was able to visualize 30 mm (15–45 mm) of LHBT compared with open subpectoral biceps tenodesis, which exposed 95 mm (75–130 mm) of LHBT. Other investigators have demonstrated similar ineptitude of diagnostic arthroscopy for visualizing the full extent of the clinical pathologic condition. Gilmer and colleagues[38] showed that diagnostic arthroscopy only identified 67% of pathologic conditions and underestimated its extent in 56% of subjects. Moon and colleagues[39] reported that 79% of proximal, arthroscopically visualized, LHBT tears propagated distally into the bicipital tunnel and were often accompanied by extensive tenosynovitis.
- In a large retrospective review of 277 subjects who underwent arthroscopic subdeltoid transfer of the LHBT to the conjoint tendon for chronic refractory BLC symptoms, lesions were categorized by location (inside, junction, and bicipital tunnel) to determine prevalence (**Fig. 6**).[1] Of this chronically symptomatic population, 47% had bicipital tunnel lesions that were concealed from standard

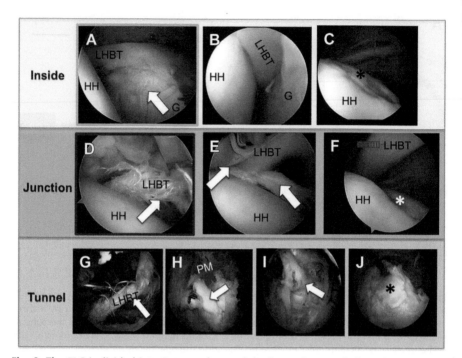

Fig. 6. The BLC is divided into 3 zones that each harbor unique pathologic lesions. Inside lesions (*A–C*) include (*A*) SLAP tears (*arrow*), (*B*) incarceration of the LHBT within the gleno-humeral joint, and (*C*) medial biceps chondromalacia, which is attritional wear of the medial humeral head from a windshield wiper effect of the LHBT (*asterisk*). Junctional lesions include (*D*) partial tears of the LHBT (*arrow*), (*E*) pulley lesion (*arrows*), and (*F*) junctional bi-ceps chondromalacia, which occurs below the LHBT near the articular margin (*asterisk*), among other lesions. Bicipital tunnel lesions are a diverse group including (*G*) partial tears (*arrow*), (*H*) loose bodies (*arrow*), (*I*) dense synovitis (*arrow*), and (*J*) extra-articular osteo-phytes (*asterisk*), among others. G, glenoid; HH, humeral head; PM, pectoralis major.

diagnostic arthroscopy. Importantly, almost half of the subjects with a junctional lesion also had a hidden tunnel lesion. The same was true for subjects with labral tears, of whom almost half also had hidden tunnel lesions.

- Sanders and colleagues[40] retrospectively looked at 127 biceps surgeries. They compared clinical failure rates between those in which the surgical technique released the extra-articular sheath and those that did not. They found a signifi-cantly higher failure rate among techniques that did not release the sheath (20.6%) than those that did (6.8%).

Long head of the biceps tendon length-tension

Regardless of the selected tenodesis location, the clinician should consider reestab-lishing the normal length-tension relationship. It is likely most important to avoid undertensioning the LHBT during tenodesis to prevent subjective sense of fatigue, discomfort, and cramping as well as an aesthetically displeasing subsidence of the bi-ceps muscle, or frank Popeye sign. Although the authors' experience suggests that overtensioning of the LHBT is less of a problem due to the muscle's dynamic ability to accommodate over time, pullout forces at the tenodesis site are increased. Thus overtensioning may increase the rate of failure.

- The LHBT distance from the origin at the supraglenoid tubercle to the articular margin is 25 to 36 mm, from the origin to the distal margin of the subscapularis tendon is 52 to 63 mm, from the origin to the proximal margin of the pectoralis major tendon is 74 to 90 mm, and from the origin to the musculotendinous junction is 99 to 138 mm.[1,22,23]
- It should be noted that the musculotendinous junction is quite variable and often begins further proximal than may be appreciated at the time of open subpectoral biceps tenodesis.[24] That being said, Jarrett and colleagues[48] found that the musculotendinous junction of the LHBT began 2.2 cm distal to the proximal margin of the pectoralis major tendon. In their cadaveric study, Lafrance and colleagues[24] reported that the musculotendinous junction began 3.2 cm distal to the proximal margin of the pectoralis major tendon and that this junction extends for an average of 7.8 cm before complete conversion to muscle, such that the junction extended for an average of 3.3 cm distal to the inferior margin of the pectoralis major tendon.

Neurovascular proximity

- During open subpectoral biceps tenodesis, external rotation of the arm increased the distance of the musculocutaneous nerve from 8.1 to 19.4 mm from the tenodesis site. Radial nerve and deep brachial artery were within 7.5 mm of the medial retractor. The median nerve, brachial artery, and brachial vein were all greater than 25 mm from the tenodesis location.[49]

Long head of the biceps tendon function
The function of the LHBT has long been a source of debate and controversy:

- Several electromyography (EMG) studies were used to evaluate muscle activation patterns during specific movements.[50–52] Levy and colleagues[53] demonstrated relative inactivity of the LHBT using indwelling thin-wire electrodes during isolated shoulder motion with the forearm and elbow maintained in a fixed position.
- Several cadaveric studies have been performed to elucidate the function of the LHBT and often conclude that it is a humeral head depressor,[54] and is important for anterior, posterior, and inferior glenohumeral stability[55–59] as well as rotational stability.[60–62] However, there are significant limitations of such biomechanical studies, particularly that they cannot account for physiologic contribution of other muscles contributing to a particular motion. More importantly, they are based on a tensioned LHBT, which is not supported by the aforementioned EMG data[53] that suggests minimal activation of the LHBT during shoulder motion.
- In perhaps the most clinically relevant study, Giphart and colleagues[63] determined the in vivo stabilizing effect of the LHBT on glenohumeral translation using 5 subjects status after open subpectoral biceps tenodesis and biplane fluoroscopy. Each individual performed a series of dynamic maneuvers under the scrutiny of biplane fluoroscopy. Each maneuver was performed using the postoperative extremity and compared with the contralateral side as an internal control. The average difference between postoperative and control side with regard to translation was less than 1.0 mm, including 0.7 mm anterior during abduction and 0.9 mm anterior during late cocking motion. The investigators concluded that subpectoral biceps tenodesis had little effect on glenohumeral kinematics.

PATHOANATOMY
Inside

- SLAP: Hwang and colleagues[64] showed that humeral head translation had a greater effect on superior glenoid labrum strain than did biceps tension. This supports the idea that SLAP tears result primarily from superior migration of the humeral head rather than biceps tension (see **Fig. 6**). Based on their cadaveric model, Patzer and colleagues[65] suggested that SLAP repair improves glenohumeral stability as long as the LHBT remains in continuity. If the biceps was tenotomized, then subsequent SLAP repair had no impact on glenohumeral translation. Strauss and colleagues[66] used a cadaveric model to demonstrate that type II SLAP tears increased glenohumeral translation in all directions and that biceps tenodesis in the setting of type II SLAP did not magnify glenohumeral instability produced by the type II SLAP tear. Although their results suggested that biceps tenodesis as a treatment for type II SLAP would not adversely impact stability, the clinician may consider concomitant superior labral repair in throwing athletes in an effort restore stability.

- LHBT incarceration (Video 1): Verma and colleagues[67] described a subset of symptomatic subjects with arthroscopically normal LHBT who had incarcerated the tendon between the glenoid and humeral head with the arm positioned in forward flexion and internal rotation (ie, mimicking the active compression test, or O'Brien sign).
- Medial biceps chondromalacia: Attritional chondral wear occurs along the anteromedial aspect of the humeral head due to the LHBT. It corresponds to the area of contact between the LHBT and humeral head during a positive arthroscopic active compression test.

Junction

- Intra-articular LHBT: Partial and complete tears of the LHBT are common, particularly along the articular margin, which is approximately 2.5 cm from the origin[22] and is a vascular watershed region.[27]
- Boileau and colleagues[68] described an hourglass biceps lesion in which the tendon hypertrophies proximal to the bicipital groove, resulting in symptoms related to entrapment of the tendon within the glenohumeral joint.
- Biceps pulley: Bennett[31] identified LHBT instability among 165 subjects undergoing shoulder arthroscopy resulting from subscapularis tears (28%) and rotator interval lesions (19%). Concomitant SLAP tears and pulley lesions are uncommon.[69] Patzer and colleagues[69] studied 182 subjects with SLAP tears (type I excluded) and 87 subjects with pulley lesions and found concomitantly occurring lesions in only 10%. History of fall onto outstretched arm predicted SLAP tear, whereas a fall with the arm in internal rotation predicted pulley lesions. Several signs of interval or pulley insufficiency have been described in the imaging literature, including displacement of the LHBT relative to the subscapularis tendon on oblique sagittal images, medial subluxation of the LHBT on axial images, discontinuity of the superior glenohumeral ligament, and the presence of biceps tendinopathy. Overall, magnetic resonance arthrography has demonstrated high sensitivities (82%–89%) and specificities (87%–98%) for pulley lesions.[70]
- Junctional biceps chondromalacia: This term, from the senior author (SJO), describes attritional wear of the humeral head below the LHBT along the articular margin. Other investigators have recognized this phenomenon. Sistermann[71] reported on "biceps tendon footprint," which was observed in 16% of 118 shoulder arthroscopies and identified a high correlation with biceps synovitis, multidirectional instability, and rotator cuff tears. Byram and colleagues[72] identified a group of subjects with humeral head abrasion below the intraarticular portion of the LHBT, and 33 of the 127 subjects in their retrospective series

had humeral head abrasions. Although this lesion was most common among subjects with failed SLAP repairs, it was also seen in the presence of other biceps pathologic conditions. Chondral lesions on the humeral head below the LHBT, called bicipital chondral prints, were observed in 78% of 182 subjects with SLAP tears (type I excluded)[73] and was independent of age or type of trauma. Furthermore, in a follow-up study, the investigators found that SLAP lesion increase anterior and anteroinferior translation and are associated with more LHBT tension.[74]

Bicipital Tunnel

Taylor and colleagues[1] recognized that the bicipital tunnel often conceals lesions from standard diagnostic arthroscopy (**Fig. 7**). In fact, they found a 47% prevalence of such lesions among 277 chronically symptomatic subjects. Gilmer and colleagues[38] noted that the bicipital tunnel concealed 33% of BLC lesions and that glenohumeral arthroscopy underestimated the magnitude of pathologic condition in 56% of cases.

- Proximally identified LHBT tears often extend distally into the bicipital tunnel. Moon and colleagues[39] recently reported that 79% of proximal, arthroscopically visualized, LHBT tears propagated distally into the bicipital tunnel and were often accompanied by extensive tenosynovitis.

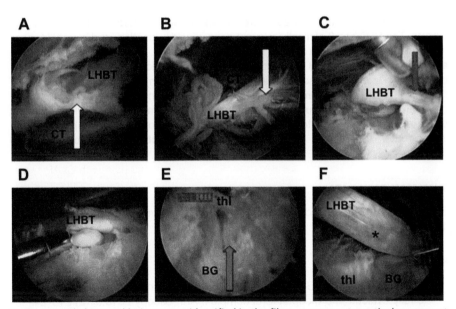

Fig. 7. Several abnormal lesions were identified in the fibro-osseous extra-articular segment of the LHBT from within the subdeltoid space during arthroscopic transfer of the LHBT to the conjoint tendon (CT), despite a normal intra-articular arthroscopic examination. Representative examples included (*A*) scarring (*white arrow*), (*B*) partial tearing (*yellow arrow*), (*C*) symptomatic vincula (*blue arrow*), (*D*) loose bodies, (*E*) bony stenosis of the bicipital groove (*red arrow*), and (*F*) instability characterized by a shallow broad osseous floor, gossamer transverse humeral ligament (thl), and resulting irritation of the LHBT (*asterisk*). BG, bicipital groove. (*From* Taylor SA, Khair MM, Gulotta LV, et al. Diagnostic glenohumeral arthroscopy fails to fully evaluate the biceps-labral complex. Arthroscopy 2015;31(2):219; with permission.)

- Numerous lesions have been described within this extra-articular space including loose bodies, scar tissue, partial LHBT tears, osseous stenosis, osteophytes, instability, synovitis, and inflamed vincula, among others.[1]
- The proximal margin of the pectoralis major defines the transition from zone 2 to zone 3 of the bicipital tunnel and is particularly important because it forms a bottleneck for many lesions, such as loose bodies and synovitis, which migrate distally but cannot decompress into the subpectoral region (zone 3). This may lead to an aggregation of space occupying lesions in zone 2 of the bicipital tunnel and produce bicipital tunnel syndrome.[1,2]
- Scar and adhesion formation in zones 1 and 2 of the bicipital tunnel are most prevalent.[1] McGahan and colleagues[26] demonstrated that such simulated adhesions produce a 47.3° loss of glenohumeral internal rotation.
- Decompression of the bicipital tunnel may be an important technical consideration in some patients. To this end, Sanders and colleagues[40] retrospectively looked at clinical failure of various biceps procedures, defined as persistent symptoms of enough severity to indicate revision surgery, in 127 shoulders. Stratification of revision rates based on surgical technique demonstrated significantly lower failure rates for procedures that released the biceps sheath (6.8%) than those that did not (20.6%).

SUMMARY

The BLC represents the shared anatomic and clinical features of the biceps and labrum. The BLC has 3 clinically relevant zones: inside, junction, and bicipital tunnel. Inside includes the superior labrum and the biceps anchor. Junction includes the intra-articular portion of the LHBT and its stabilizing pulley, which is visualized during standard glenohumeral arthroscopy. Bicipital tunnel represents the extra-articular LHBT from the articular margin through the subpectoral region and its fibro-osseous confinement termed the bicipital tunnel. Embracing this more comprehensive understanding of the anatomy, pathoanatomy, and functional implications, clinicians can proceed with greater confidence and more accurately select patient-specific surgical techniques.

SUPPLEMENTARY DATA

Supplementary data related to this article can be found online at http://dx.doi.org/10.1016/j.csm.2015.08.005.

REFERENCES

1. Taylor SA, Khair MM, Gulotta LV, et al. Diagnostic glenohumeral arthroscopy fails to fully evaluate the biceps-labral complex. Arthroscopy 2015;31(2):215–24.
2. Taylor SA, Fabricant PD, Bansal M, et al. The anatomy and histology of the bicipital tunnel of the shoulder. J Shoulder Elbow Surg 2015;24(4):511–9.
3. Cooper DE, Arnoczky SP, O'Brien SJ, et al. Anatomy, histology, and vascularity of the glenoid labrum. An anatomical study. J Bone Joint Surg Am 1992;74(1):46–52.
4. Prescher A. Anatomical basics, variations, and degenerative changes of the shoulder joint and shoulder girdle. Eur J Radiol 2000;35(2):88–102.
5. O'Brien SJ, Neves MC, Arnoczky SP, et al. The anatomy and histology of the inferior glenohumeral ligament complex of the shoulder. Am J Sports Med 1990;18(5):449–56.

6. Ilahi OA, Labbe MR, Cosculluela P. Variants of the anterosuperior glenoid labrum and associated pathology. Arthroscopy 2002;18(8):882–6.

7. Pfahler M, Haraida S, Schulz C, et al. Age-related changes of the glenoid labrum in normal shoulders. J Shoulder Elbow Surg 2003;12(1):40–52.

8. Williams MM, Snyder SJ, Buford D Jr. The Buford complex—the "cord-like" middle glenohumeral ligament and absent anterosuperior labrum complex: a normal anatomic capsulolabral variant. Arthroscopy 1994;10(3):241–7.

9. Ide J, Maeda S, Takagi K. Normal variations of the glenohumeral ligament complex: an anatomic study for arthroscopic Bankart repair. Arthroscopy 2004;20(2): 164–8.

10. Cawley PW, Heidt RS Jr, Scranton PE Jr, et al. Physiologic axial load, frictional resistance, and the football shoe-surface interface. Foot Ankle Int 2003;24(7): 551–6.

11. Tuoheti Y, Itoi E, Minagawa H, et al. Attachment types of the long head of the biceps tendon to the glenoid labrum and their relationships with the glenohumeral ligaments. Arthroscopy 2005;21(10):1242–9.

12. Hootman JM, Dick R, Agel J. Epidemiology of collegiate injuries for 15 sports: summary and recommendations for injury prevention initiatives. J Athl Train 2007;42(2):311–9.

13. Arai R, Mochizuki T, Yamaguchi K, et al. Functional anatomy of the superior glenohumeral and coracohumeral ligaments and the subscapularis tendon in view of stabilization of the long head of the biceps tendon. J Shoulder Elbow Surg 2010; 19(1):58–64.

14. Rispoli DM, Athwal GS, Sperling JW, et al. The macroscopic delineation of the edge of the glenoid labrum: an anatomic evaluation of an open and arthroscopic visual reference. Arthroscopy 2009;25(6):603–7.

15. Connell DA, Potter HG, Wickiewicz TL, et al. Noncontrast magnetic resonance imaging of superior labral lesions. 102 cases confirmed at arthroscopic surgery. Am J Sports Med 1999;27(2):208–13.

16. Vangsness CT Jr, Jorgenson SS, Watson T, et al. The origin of the long head of the biceps from the scapula and glenoid labrum. An anatomical study of 100 shoulders. J Bone Joint Surg Br 1994;76(6):951–4.

17. Pal GP, Bhatt RH, Patel VS. Relationship between the tendon of the long head of biceps brachii and the glenoidal labrum in humans. Anat Rec 1991;229(2): 278–80.

18. Dierickx C, Ceccarelli E, Conti M, et al. Variations of the intra-articular portion of the long head of the biceps tendon: a classification of embryologically explained variations. J Shoulder Elbow Surg 2009;18(4):556–65.

19. Franco JC, Knapp TP, Mandelbaum BR. Congenital absence of the long head of the biceps tendon. A case report. J Bone Joint Surg Am 2005;87(7):1584–6.

20. Hyman JL, Warren RF. Extra-articular origin of biceps brachii. Arthroscopy 2001; 17(7):E29.

21. Wahl CJ, MacGillivray JD. Three congenital variations in the long head of the biceps tendon: a review of pathoanatomic considerations and case reports. J Shoulder Elbow Surg 2007;16(6):e25–30.

22. Denard PJ, Dai X, Hanypsiak BT, et al. Anatomy of the biceps tendon: implications for restoring physiological length-tension relation during biceps tenodesis with interference screw fixation. Arthroscopy 2012;28(10):1352–8.

23. Hussain WM, Reddy D, Atanda A, et al. The longitudinal anatomy of the long head of the biceps tendon and implications on tenodesis. Knee Surg Sports Traumatol Arthrosc 2015;23(5):1518–23.

24. Lafrance R, Madsen W, Yaseen Z, et al. Relevant anatomic landmarks and measurements for biceps tenodesis. Am J Sports Med 2013;41(6):1395–9.

25. Braun S, Horan MP, Elser F, et al. Lesions of the biceps pulley. Am J Sports Med 2011;39(4):790–5.

26. McGahan PJ, Patel H, Dickinson E, et al. The effect of biceps adhesions on glenohumeral range of motion: a cadaveric study. J Shoulder Elbow Surg 2013; 22(5):658–65.

27. Cheng NM, Pan WR, Vally F, et al. The arterial supply of the long head of biceps tendon: Anatomical study with implications for tendon rupture. Clin Anat 2010; 23(6):683–92.

28. Alpantaki K, McLaughlin D, Karagogeos D, et al. Sympathetic and sensory neural elements in the tendon of the long head of the biceps. J Bone Joint Surg Am 2005;87(7):1580–3.

29. Alpantaki K, Savvaki M, Karagogeos D. Expression of cell adhesion molecule L1 in the long head of biceps tendon. Cell Mol Biol (Noisy-le-grand) 2010;56(Suppl): OL1286–9.

30. Tosounidis T, Hadjileontis C, Triantafyllou C, et al. Evidence of sympathetic innervation and alpha1-adrenergic receptors of the long head of the biceps brachii tendon. J Orthop Sci 2013;18(2):238–44.

31. Bennett WF. Visualization of the anatomy of the rotator interval and bicipital sheath. Arthroscopy 2001;17(1):107–11.

32. Hart ND, Golish SR, Dragoo JL. Effects of arm position on maximizing intra-articular visualization of the biceps tendon: a cadaveric study. Arthroscopy 2012;28(4):481–5.

33. Habermeyer P, Magosch P, Pritsch M, et al. Anterosuperior impingement of the shoulder as a result of pulley lesions: a prospective arthroscopic study. J Shoulder Elbow Surg 2004;13(1):5–12.

34. Kask K, Poldoja E, Lont T, et al. Anatomy of the superior glenohumeral ligament. J Shoulder Elbow Surg 2010;19(6):908–16.

35. Yeh L, Kwak S, Kim YS, et al. Anterior labroligamentous structures of the glenohumeral joint: correlation of MR arthrography and anatomic dissection in cadavers. AJR Am J Roentgenol 1998;171(5):1229–36.

36. Braun S, Millett PJ, Yongpravat C, et al. Biomechanical evaluation of shear force vectors leading to injury of the biceps reflection pulley: a biplane fluoroscopy study on cadaveric shoulders. Am J Sports Med 2010;38(5):1015–24.

37. Festa A, Allert J, Issa K, et al. Visualization of the extra-articular portion of the long head of the biceps tendon during intra-articular shoulder arthroscopy. Arthroscopy 2014;30(11):1413–7.

38. Gilmer BB, DeMers AM, Guerrero D, et al. Arthroscopic versus open comparison of long head of biceps tendon visualization and pathology in patients requiring tenodesis. Arthroscopy 2015;31(1):29–34.

39. Moon SC, Cho NS, Rhee YG. Analysis of "hidden lesions" of the extra-articular biceps after subpectoral biceps tenodesis: the subpectoral portion as the optimal tenodesis site. Am J Sports Med 2015;43(1):63–8.

40. Sanders B, Lavery KP, Pennington S, et al. Clinical success of biceps tenodesis with and without release of the transverse humeral ligament. J Shoulder Elbow Surg 2012;21(1):66–71.

41. Pfahler M, Branner S, Refior HJ. The role of the bicipital groove in tendopathy of the long biceps tendon. J Shoulder Elbow Surg 1999;8(5):419–24.

42. Cone RO, Danzig L, Resnick D, et al. The bicipital groove: radiographic, anatomic, and pathologic study. AJR Am J Roentgenol 1983;141(4):781–8.

43. Gleason PD, Beall DP, Sanders TG, et al. The transverse humeral ligament: a separate anatomical structure or a continuation of the osseous attachment of the rotator cuff? Am J Sports Med 2006;34(1):72–7.
44. MacDonald K, Bridger J, Cash C, et al. Transverse humeral ligament: does it exist? Clin Anat 2007;20(6):663–7.
45. Romeo AA, Mazzocca AD, Tauro JC. Arthroscopic biceps tenodesis. Arthroscopy 2004;20(2):206–13.
46. Burkhead WZ, Habermeyer P, Walch G, et al. Chapter 26: the biceps tendon. In: Rockwood CA, Wirth MA, Matsen FA, et al, editors. The shoulder, 4th edition. Philadelphia: Saunders Elsevier; 2009. p. 1309–60.
47. Yamaguchi K, Riew KD, Galatz LM, et al. Biceps activity during shoulder motion: an electromyographic analysis. Clin Orthop Relat Res 1997;(336):122–9.
48. Jarrett CD, McClelland WB Jr, Xerogeanes JW. Minimally invasive proximal biceps tenodesis: an anatomical study for optimal placement and safe surgical technique. J Shoulder Elbow Surg 2011;20(3):477–80.
49. Dickens JF, Kilcoyne KG, Tintle SM, et al. Subpectoral biceps tenodesis: an anatomic study and evaluation of at-risk structures. Am J Sports Med 2012; 40(10):2337–41.
50. Escamilla RF, Andrews JR. Shoulder muscle recruitment patterns and related biomechanics during upper extremity sports. Sports Med 2009;39(7):569–90.
51. Kelly BT, Backus SI, Warren RF, et al. Electromyographic analysis and phase definition of the overhead football throw. Am J Sports Med 2002;30(6):837–44.
52. Ryu RK, McCormick J, Jobe FW, et al. An electromyographic analysis of shoulder function in tennis players. Am J Sports Med 1988;16(5):481–5.
53. Levy AS, Kelly BT, Lintner SA, et al. Function of the long head of the biceps at the shoulder: electromyographic analysis. J Shoulder Elbow Surg 2001;10(3): 250–5.
54. Kumar VP, Satku K, Balasubramaniam P. The role of the long head of biceps brachii in the stabilization of the head of the humerus. Clin Orthop Relat Res 1989;(244):172–5.
55. Blasier RB, Soslowsky LJ, Malicky DM, et al. Posterior glenohumeral subluxation: active and passive stabilization in a biomechanical model. J Bone Joint Surg Am 1997;79(3):433–40.
56. Itoi E, Kuechle DK, Newman SR, et al. Stabilising function of the biceps in stable and unstable shoulders. J Bone Joint Surg Br 1993;75(4):546–50.
57. Itoi E, Newman SR, Kuechle DK, et al. Dynamic anterior stabilisers of the shoulder with the arm in abduction. J Bone Joint Surg Br 1994;76(5):834–6.
58. Pagnani MJ, Deng XH, Warren RF, et al. Role of the long head of the biceps brachii in glenohumeral stability: a biomechanical study in cadavera. J Shoulder Elbow Surg 1996;5(4):255–62.
59. Soslowsky LJ, Malicky DM, Blasier RB. Active and passive factors in inferior glenohumeral stabilization: a biomechanical model. J Shoulder Elbow Surg 1997; 6(4):371–9.
60. Youm T, ElAttrache NS, Tibone JE, et al. The effect of the long head of the biceps on glenohumeral kinematics. J Shoulder Elbow Surg 2009;18(1):122–9.
61. Rodosky MW, Harner CD, Fu FH. The role of the long head of the biceps muscle and superior glenoid labrum in anterior stability of the shoulder. Am J Sports Med 1994;22(1):121–30.
62. Kuhn JE, Huston LJ, Soslowsky LJ, et al. External rotation of the glenohumeral joint: ligament restraints and muscle effects in the neutral and abducted positions. J Shoulder Elbow Surg 2005;14(1 Suppl S):39S–48S.

63. Giphart JE, Elser F, Dewing CB, et al. The long head of the biceps tendon has minimal effect on in vivo glenohumeral kinematics: a biplane fluoroscopy study. Am J Sports Med 2012;40(1):202–12.

64. Hwang E, Carpenter JE, Hughes RE, et al. Effects of biceps tension and superior humeral head translation on the glenoid labrum. J Orthop Res 2014;32(11): 1424–9.

65. Patzer T, Habermeyer P, Hurschler C, et al. The influence of superior labrum anterior to posterior (SLAP) repair on restoring baseline glenohumeral translation and increased biceps loading after simulated SLAP tear and the effectiveness of SLAP repair after long head of biceps tenotomy. J Shoulder Elbow Surg 2012; 21(11):1580–7.

66. Strauss EJ, Salata MJ, Sershon RA, et al. Role of the superior labrum after biceps tenodesis in glenohumeral stability. J Shoulder Elbow Surg 2014;23(4):485–91.

67. Verma NN, Drakos M, O'Brien SJ. The arthroscopic active compression test. Arthroscopy 2005;21(5):634.

68. Boileau P, Ahrens PM, Trojani C, et al. Entrapment of the long head of the biceps: the "hourglass biceps". Another cause of pain and locking of the shoulder. Rev Chir Orthop Reparatrice Appar Mot 2003;89(8):672–82.

69. Patzer T, Kircher J, Lichtenberg S, et al. Is there an association between SLAP lesions and biceps pulley lesions? Arthroscopy 2011;27(5):611–8.

70. Schaeffeler C, Waldt S, Holzapfel K, et al. Lesions of the biceps pulley: diagnostic accuracy of MR arthrography of the shoulder and evaluation of previously described and new diagnostic signs. Radiology 2012;264(2):504–13.

71. Sistermann R. The biceps tendon footprint. Acta Orthop 2005;76(2):237–40.

72. Byram IR, Dunn WR, Kuhn JE. Humeral head abrasion: an association with failed superior labrum anterior posterior repairs. J Shoulder Elbow Surg 2011;20(1): 92–7.

73. Patzer T, Lichtenberg S, Kircher J, et al. Influence of SLAP lesions on chondral lesions of the glenohumeral joint. Knee Surg Sports Traumatol Arthrosc 2010; 18(7):982–7.

74. Patzer T, Habermeyer P, Hurschler C, et al. Increased glenohumeral translation and biceps load after SLAP lesions with potential influence on glenohumeral chondral lesions: a biomechanical study on human cadavers. Knee Surg Sports Traumatol Arthrosc 2011;19(10):1780–7.

Injuries to the Biceps Pulley

Frank Martetschläger, MD, PhD[a,b,*], Mark Tauber, MD, PhD[a,c],
Peter Habermeyer, Prof, MD[a]

KEYWORDS

- Biceps reflection pulley • Pulley lesions • Biceps tendon injuries • Biceps instability

KEY POINTS

- The biceps reflection pulley (BRP) is a capsuloligamentous complex acting to stabilize the long head of the biceps tendon (LHB) before it enters the bicipital groove.
- Injuries to the biceps pulley contribute to instability of the LHB.
- The unstable and inflamed LHB may lead to painful impairment of shoulder function.
- In most cases, surgical intervention is required to treat biceps pulley lesions and different surgical options exist.
- Tenotomy or tenodesis of the LHB seems most reliable.

INTRODUCTION

The BRP is a soft tissue sling consisting of fibers of the superior glenohumeral ligament (SGHL), the coracohumeral ligament (CHL), and the supraspinatus tendon (SSP) and subscapularis tendon (SSC) (**Fig. 1**). It acts to stabilize the tendon course of the LHB before it enters the bony bicipital groove.[1,2] Acute trauma, repetitive microtrauma, and degeneration of the involved soft tissues can result in a lesion of the biceps pulley.[3–5] The prevalence of BRP lesions during shoulder arthroscopy is 7%, rendering this lesion a common pathology and a considerable source of morbidity.[3] Injuries to the BRP with concomitant painful instability of the LHB are often found in patients with anterior shoulder pain.[4] Several studies have shown the LHB to act as an important pain generator inside the shoulder joint, which is due to the profuse innervation of the proximal third of the tendon.[6–8] Injuries to the BRP are associated with tears of

Disclaimer: None of the authors has any conflict of interest to declare regarding this article. One or more of the authors are paid/unpaid consultants for Arthrex.
[a] Deutsches Schulterzentrum, ATOS Clinic Munich, Effnerstraße 38, Munich 81925, Germany; [b] Department of Orthopaedic Sports Medicine, Klinikum rechts der Isar, Technical University Munich, Munich, Germany; [c] Department of Traumatology and Sports Injuries, Paracelsus Medical University, Salzburg, Austria
* Corresponding author. Deutsches Schulterzentrum, ATOS Clinic Munich, Effnerstraße 38, Munich 81925, Germany.
E-mail address: martetschlaeger@atos-muenchen.de

http://dx.doi.org/10.1016/j.csm.2015.08.003
0278-5919/16/$ – see front matter © 2016 Elsevier Inc. All rights reserved.
sportsmed.theclinics.com

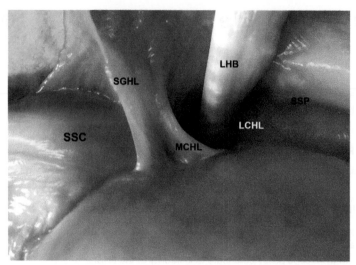

Fig. 1. Anatomy of the BRP in a cadaveric shoulder. LCHL, lateral CHL; MCHL, medial CHL.

the rotator cuff, superior labrum anterior-posterior lesions, biceps instability, and biceps tears.[4,9–12] Furthermore, BRP lesions have been reported associated with an internal anterosuperior impingement.[13] Several studies have published different classification systems for LHB dislocation or subluxation.[7,9,12,13] There is still little information in the literature, however, regarding the pathomechanism of BRP injuries. In a fluoroscopy study, Braun and colleagues[14] reported that increased shear forces at forward flexion with neutral or internal arm rotation and internal rotation at normal arm position may cause injury to the BRP. Classification systems, clinical and radiographic presentation, and arthroscopic evaluation are described along with the current treatment options.

CLASSIFICATION

Bennett's[9] classification system subdivides BRP lesions based on the anatomic structure injured. In cases of an intra-articular subscapularis lesion (type 1) or if the medial head of the CHL is incompetent (type 2), the biceps tendon displays increased intra-sheath mobility. When both the subscapularis and medial head of the CHL are disrupted, the biceps dislocates intra-articularly (type 3). A lesion of the lateral CHL along with a leading edge injury of the subscapularis may lead to dislocation of the LHB anterior to the subscapularis (type 4). When each structure is disrupted, complete loss of integrity of the bicipital sheath occurs (type 5).[9]

In 2004, Habermeyer and colleagues[13] identified and described 4 different groups of pulley lesions and established a new classification system. Group 1 lesions represent isolated lesions of the SGHL. If the SGHL is injured along with an articular-sided SSP or SSC tear, the lesion is classified into groups 2 and 3. Group 4 is a combination of the described lesions (**Fig. 2**).

CLINICAL EXAMINATION

Clinical diagnosis of lesions to the biceps pulley is difficult because these lesions are often associated with pathology of the surrounding tissue, especially the rotator cuff tendons of the supraspinatus and subscapularis. Therefore, no specific test for pulley

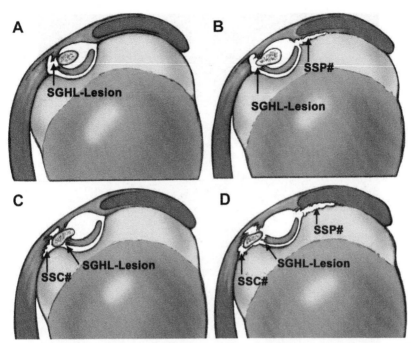

Fig. 2. Habermeyer classification of BRP lesions. (*From* Habermeyer P, Magosch P, Pritsch M, et al. Anterosuperior impingement of the shoulder as a result of pulley lesions: a prospective arthroscopic study. J Shoulder Elbow Surg 2004;13:5–12; with permission.)

lesions has been described. In 89 patients with pulley lesions, Habermeyer and colleagues[13] found a positive impingement sign in 53% and a positive palm up or O'Brien test in 66% of the patients. Because instability of the biceps tendon may result in inflammation of the tendon, literally all biceps tests can be positive during examination. Ben Kibler and colleagues[15] recommended a combination of the Speed's test and upper cut test to detect biceps pathology. This study has not investigated, however, pulley lesions specifically. These data emphasize that further investigation is necessary regarding the optimal clinical examination of injuries to the biceps pulley.

IMAGING

Several studies have suggested magnetic resonance (MR) arthrography as the best option for detection of pulley lesions.[3,16,17] Walch and colleagues[18] described the pulley sign as an extra-articular collection of contrast material anterior to the superior extent of the subscapularis. Its presence on MR arthrography studies suggests a lesion to the BRP. Also, the extension of contrast to the cortex of the coracoid may be helpful in the preoperative diagnosis of rotator interval lesions.[19] A recent study by Schaeffeler and colleagues[20] investigated the diagnostic accuracy of MR arthrography for detection of pulley lesions and evaluated previously described and new diagnostic signs. They found that MR arthrography was accurate in the detection of pulley lesions, with the displacement sign, the nonvisibility or discontinuity of the SGHL, and tendinopathy of the LHB on oblique sagittal images the most accurate criteria (**Fig. 3**). Therefore, for evaluation of the BRP, a T1-weighted MR arthrography should be obtained and clinicians should be aware of the critical signs.

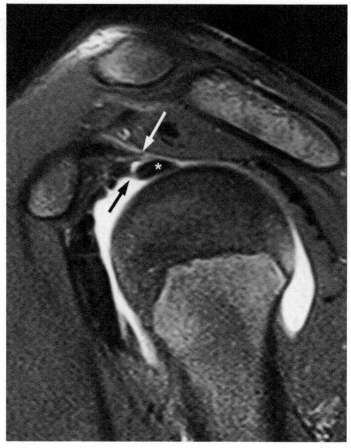

Fig. 3. Normal anatomy of the BRP on a sagittal, fat-saturated, T1-weighted MR arthrography. LHB (*asterisk*), CHL (*white arrow*), and SGHL (*black arrow*).

INDICATIONS FOR OPERATIVE TREATMENT

After a lesion to the BRP is diagnosed, surgical treatment is indicated after a course of failed conservative treatment. In daily clinical practice, conservative treatment with anti-inflammatory drugs and physiotherapy seems to fail in most cases of BRP lesions. This might be due to persistent LHB instability maintaining recurrent pain and impairment of shoulder function. Higher-grade lesions of the BRP with concomitant lesions of the rotator cuff should also be considered for surgical treatment, especially in younger patients.

SURGICAL OPTIONS

Surgical options for the treatment of BRP lesions comprise open or arthroscopic repair and tenotomy or tenodesis of the LHB. Because clinical results suggest that tenotomy and tenodesis provide more reliable outcomes, most shoulder surgeons favor these procedures over BRP repair. In young and active patients, especially athletes, the authors recommend that surgeons perform a biceps tenodesis. In older patients without significant cosmetic concerns, simple tenotomy is sufficient treatment.

Preparation and Patient Positioning

Only standard arthroscopic instruments are necessary. In cases of biceps tenodesis, a biotenodesis screw or button might be necessary, depending on the desired technique. The patient is placed in the beach chair position and the injured shoulder is prepped freely in a standard fashion, allowing for free movement of the arm during surgery. The bony landmarks are marked on the skin.

Diagnostic Arthroscopy

Diagnostic arthroscopy is performed by use of a standard 30° scope through the posterior viewing portal. The scope is advanced into the anterior compartment, and the structures of the BRP are thoroughly investigated under direct visualization. Motion analysis with the arm rotating internally and externally can help evaluate stability of the LHB or demonstrate loosening of the BRP. The LHB is then pulled into the joint by use of a probe to examine the proximal part of the extra-articular portion, which might show signs of peritendinitis. The rotator cuff should be assessed carefully during motion of the shoulder (especially internal rotation for subscapularis and external rotation/abduction for supraspinatus) to not to miss hidden lesions. A normal BRP system is shown in **Fig. 4**. **Figs. 5** and **6** display common types of pulley lesions.

THE AUTHORS' PREFERRED TECHNIQUE FOR TREATMENT OF BICEPS PULLEY LESIONS

The authors' preference is to perform a tenotomy or suprapectoral biceps tenodesis in patients with lesions to the BRP. The authors think these 2 techniques are more reliable treatment options compared with the BRP repair.

For both techniques, a standard posterior viewing portal is used along with a standard anterosuperior portal through the rotator interval. For biceps tenodesis, a second suprabicipital working portal is established directly anterior to the biceps tendon, whereas the correct position should be evaluated by use of a spinal needle. The biceps tendon is then cut at its base through the anterosuperior portal with an arthroscopic scissor. The tendon slides into the bony channel where it heals in. If a portion of the tendon stump remains intra-articular, it is resected with a shaver. When performing a tenodesis, the tendon is fixed with a clamp and can be exteriorized through the biceps working portal after tenotomy. No. 2 permanent suture is then placed along its proximal 1.5 cm in a whipstitch fashion while the intra-articular portion is cut off. A drill is used to fashion a tunnel approximately 20 mm in depth at the

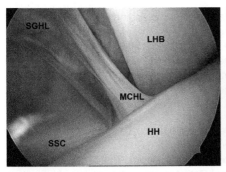 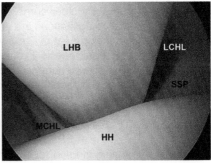

Fig. 4. Normal arthroscopic anatomy of the BRP. HH, humeral head; LCHL, lateral CHL; LHB, long head of biceps tendon; MCHL, medial CHL; SGHL, superior glenohumeral ligament; SSC, subscapularis tendon.

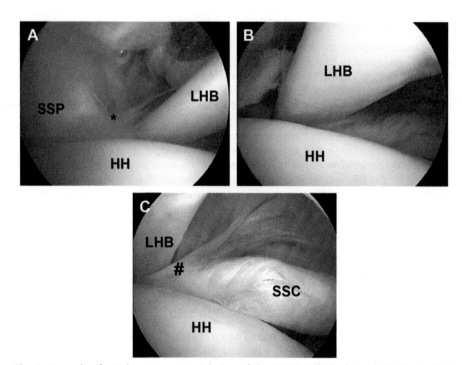

Fig. 5. Example of a Habermeyer type 2 lesion of the BRP. (*A, B*) The lateral CHL (*asterisk*) is disrupted and the SSP shows a partial lesion. (*C*) The medial BRP sling is intact (*hashtag*).

proximal aspect of the bicipital groove. Care must be taken to ensure correct tunnel placement in the center of the humerus. A bioabsorbable screw (eg, BioComposite SwiveLock, Arthrex, Naples, Florida) is loaded with 1 strand of the suture and used to fix the tendon within the bone tunnel and advanced until it is flush with the humeral cortex. The 2 ends of the suture are tied over the screw, enhancing screw-tendon security. **Fig. 7** shows the crucial steps of the procedure.

COMPLICATIONS AND MANAGEMENT

The complications related to this procedure are standard complications, as known with any arthroscopic shoulder surgery, and involve bleeding, joint infection, and nerve injury. Special complications are ongoing pain in the biceps region or cramping of the muscle, development of Popeye deformity and retearing of the tendon out of the bony socket after tenodesis. In cases of retearing of the tendon, a subpectoral biceps tenodesis can be performed through a mini–open approach according to patients' wishes and expectations, whereby the authors' recommendation is restrictive.

POSTOPERATIVE CARE

Postoperatively, a sling is used for no longer than 2 weeks. The rehabilitation plan varies according to concomitant procedures. Resisted elbow flexion is not permitted for 6 weeks. In isolated BRP lesions without need for rotator cuff surgery, passive glenohumeral and elbow motion should begin immediately and advance to active motion

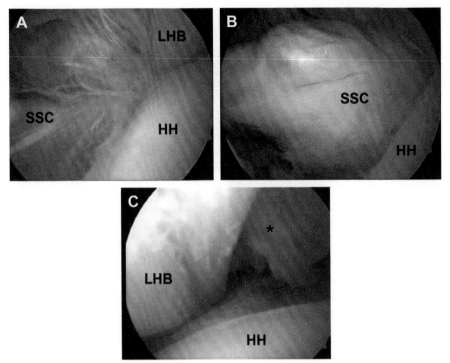

Fig. 6. Example of a Habermeyer type 4 lesion of the BRP. (*A, B*) The medial CHL is disrupted and the SSC shows a partial lesion. (*C*) SGHL is disrupted (*asterisk*) and SSP is torn.

as the patient tolerates. Strengthening or heavy weight lifting should be withheld for 6 weeks.

OUTCOMES

Lesions of the BRP can be repaired surgically, but results are mixed. Walch and colleagues[18] investigated open subscapularis reattachment and medial biceps sheath reconstruction; 12 of 22 patients required scar removal or groove deepening to stabilize an enlarged tendon. The authors found tendon rupture in 3 patients and modest pain improvement, therefore concluding that biceps tenodesis is a more reliable treatment option. Bennett[21] advocated for an arthroscopic repair technique and reported significant pain relief and improvement of shoulder function at 2-year follow-up. Repair of the BRP, however, has not gained widespread acceptance as an effective procedure among shoulder surgeons.[4,5] Literature reports good and reliable surgical outcomes after tenotomy or tenodesis for lesions to the LHB.[22] A recent meta-analysis reported no significant differences regarding the functional outcome between tenotomy and tenodesis for the treatment of LHB lesions. Popeye deformity and cramping has been shown to occur in 26% of the patients after tenotomy, which was significantly more often compared with the tenodesis group, which demonstrated a rate of 16%.[23] There is no specific analysis in the current literature investigating the outcome after tenotomy or tenodesis for the treatment of injuries to the BRP.

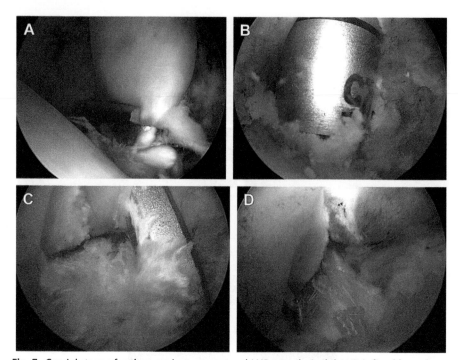

Fig. 7. Crucial steps of arthroscopic suprapectoral LHB tenodesis. (*A*) LHB is fixed by a clamp and exteriorized through the suprabicipital portal after tenotomy. (*B*) For most cases, a 6-mm bone tunnel is drilled, approximately 20 mm in depth. (*C*) One of the whipstitch sutures is then loaded in the eyelet of a 6.25-mm SwiveLock anchor and the anchor (Arthrex Inc, Naples, FL, USA) is inserted into the tunnel while tensioning the suture. (*D*) Correct and stable fixation is examined using a probe.

SUMMARY

Injuries to the BRP lead to instability of the LHB and represent a relevant source of anterior shoulder pain. The lesions are classified depending on the structures involved. In cases of unsuccessful conservative treatment, surgical management needs to be considered. Options for surgical treatment comprise open or arthroscopic repair of the BRP and tenotomy or tenodesis of the LHB. Although comparative studies are lacking in the literature, tenotomy or tenodesis of the LHB seems a more reliable procedure in the hands of most shoulder surgeons.

REFERENCES

1. Gohlke F, Essigkrug B, Schmitz F. The pattern of the collagen fiber bundles of the capsule of the glenohumeral joint. J Shoulder Elbow Surg 1994;3(3):111–28.
2. Werner A, Mueller T, Boehm D, et al. The stabilizing sling for the long head of the biceps tendon in the rotator cuff interval. A histoanatomic study. Am J Sports Med 2000;28(1):28–31.
3. Baumann B, Genning K, Böhm D, et al. Arthroscopic prevalence of pulley lesions in 1007 consecutive patients. J Shoulder Elbow Surg 2008;17(1):14–20.
4. Braun S, Horan MP, Elser F, et al. Lesions of the biceps pulley. Am J Sports Med 2011;39(4):790–5.

5. Gaskill TR, Braun S, Millett PJ. Multimedia article. The rotator interval: pathology and management. Arthroscopy 2011;27(4):556–67.
6. Curtis AS, Snyder SJ. Evaluation and treatment of biceps tendon pathology. Orthop Clin North Am 1993;24(1):33–43.
7. Szabo I, Boileau P, Walch G. The proximal biceps as a pain generator and results of tenotomy. Sports Med Arthrosc 2008;16(3):180–6.
8. Alpantaki K, McLaughlin D, Karagogeos D, et al. Sympathetic and sensory neural elements in the tendon of the long head of the biceps. J Bone Joint Surg Am 2005;87(7):1580–3.
9. Bennett WF. Arthroscopic repair of anterosuperior (supraspinatus/subscapularis) rotator cuff tears: a prospective cohort with 2- to 4-year follow-up. Classification of biceps subluxation/instability. Arthroscopy 2003;19(1):21–33.
10. Bennett WF. Subscapularis, medial, and lateral head coracohumeral ligament insertion anatomy. Arthroscopic appearance and incidence of "hidden" rotator interval lesions. Arthroscopy 2001;17(2):173–80.
11. Collier SG, Wynn-Jones CH. Displacement of the biceps with subscapularis avulsion. J Bone Joint Surg Br 1990;72(1):145.
12. Walch G, Nové-Josserand L, Boileau P, et al. Subluxations and dislocations of the tendon of the long head of the biceps. J Shoulder Elbow Surg 1998;7(2):100–8.
13. Habermeyer P, Magosch P, Pritsch M, et al. Anterosuperior impingement of the shoulder as a result of pulley lesions: a prospective arthroscopic study. J Shoulder Elbow Surg 2004;13(1):5–12.
14. Braun S, Millett PJ, Yongpravat C, et al. Biomechanical evaluation of shear force vectors leading to injury of the biceps reflection pulley: a biplane fluoroscopy study on cadaveric shoulders. Am J Sports Med 2010;38(5):1015–24.
15. Ben Kibler W, Sciascia AD, Hester P, et al. Clinical utility of traditional and new tests in the diagnosis of biceps tendon injuries and superior labrum anterior and posterior lesions in the shoulder. Am J Sports Med 2009;37(9):1840–7.
16. Bennett WF. Specificity of the Speed's test: arthroscopic technique for evaluating the biceps tendon at the level of the bicipital groove. Arthroscopy 1998;14(8):789–96.
17. Chung CB, Dwek JR, Cho GJ, et al. Rotator cuff interval: evaluation with MR imaging and MR arthrography of the shoulder in 32 cadavers. J Comput Assist Tomogr 2000;24(5):738–43.
18. Walch G, Nove-Josserand L, Levigne C, et al. Tears of the supraspinatus tendon associated with "hidden" lesions of the rotator interval. J Shoulder Elbow Surg 1994;3(6):353–60.
19. Vinson EN, Major NM, Higgins LD. Magnetic resonance imaging findings associated with surgically proven rotator interval lesions. Skeletal Radiol 2007;36(5):405–10.
20. Schaeffeler C, Waldt S, Holzapfel K, et al. Lesions of the biceps pulley: diagnostic accuracy of MR arthrography of the shoulder and evaluation of previously described and new diagnostic signs. Radiology 2012;264(2):504–13.
21. Bennett WF. Arthroscopic bicipital sheath repair: two-year follow-up with pulley lesions. Arthroscopy 2004;20(9):964–73.
22. Delle Rose G, Borroni M, Silvestro A, et al. The long head of biceps as a source of pain in active population: tenotomy or tenodesis? A comparison of 2 case series with isolated lesions. Musculoskelet Surg 2012;96(Suppl 1):S47–52.
23. Gurnani N, van Deurzen DF, Janmaat VT, et al. Tenotomy or tenodesis for pathology of the long head of the biceps brachii: a systematic review and meta-analysis. Knee Surg Sports Traumatol Arthrosc 2015. [Epub ahead of print].

Examination of the Biceps Tendon

Edward G. McFarland, MD[a],*, Amrut Borade, MD[b]

KEYWORDS

- Biceps tendon • Examination • Labrum • Range of motion • Rotator cuff • Shoulder
- Strength

KEY POINTS

- A variety of biceps tendon abnormalities can contribute to pain in the shoulder.
- There is no single pattern of pain that distinguishes biceps conditions from other shoulder abnormalities.
- Physical examination tests for biceps lesions and superior labrum anterior and posterior lesions rarely have both high sensitivity and specificity.

INTRODUCTION

The role of the long head of the biceps tendon in producing shoulder symptoms has been contested for more than 100 years. However, there is general agreement that lesions of the long head of the biceps tendon can contribute to symptoms of pain and clicking in the shoulder. This conclusion is based on the observation that before the rupture of the long head of the biceps tendon, many patients have substantial shoulder pain (mostly anteriorly), which is relieved when the tendon completely tears and retracts distally in the arm. In most patients, after the tendon tears the shoulder pain resolves, suggesting that the long head of the biceps was the origin of the pain.

The physical examination of the shoulder for lesions of the long head of the biceps is challenging for several reasons. First, there is no one pain pattern distinctive for long head of the biceps abnormalities. Further, there have been no studies in which the biceps tendon sheath was injected with an irritant to define the pain pattern. Similarly, studies of various shoulder abnormalities have shown that most lesions in this area,

Disclosure statement: no financial interests.
[a] Division of Shoulder and Elbow Surgery, Department of Orthopaedic Surgery, The Johns Hopkins University, 10753 Falls Road, Pavilion II, Suite 215, Lutherville, Baltimore, MD 21093, USA;
[b] Division of Shoulder and Elbow Surgery, Department of Orthopaedic Surgery, The Johns Hopkins University, 601 North Caroline Street, Baltimore, MD 21287, USA
* Corresponding author.
E-mail address: emacfarl1@jhmi.edu

including those involving the acromioclavicular joint, can present as pain in various locations.[1,2]

Although patients often say they have biceps pain and point to the upper part of the biceps muscle, that pain could actually be referred from a variety of shoulder abnormalities. These include rotator cuff syndrome, osteoarthritis, adhesive capsulitis, shoulder instability, and even acromioclavicular disorders.[2] Previous studies have shown a high rate of coexisting shoulder lesions in the presence of biceps tendon abnormality. Murthi and colleagues[3] found that, among patients operated on for impingement syndrome, 40% had biceps tendon abnormalities and 91% had rotator cuff tears. In their biceps tenosynovectomy group, partial-thickness rotator cuff tears were present in 47% of cases and full-thickness rotator cuff tears were present in 23%. Chen and colleagues[4] reported that 41% of 122 patients with rotator cuff tears had a variety of biceps tendon abnormalities. In patients with a large or massive rotator cuff tear, 92% had biceps tendon lesions and 97% of patients with subscapularis tendon abnormality had concomitant biceps tendon abnormality.[4] Because of these high reported rates of biceps lesions associated with other shoulder abnormalities, it is difficult to determine if the findings on examination of the shoulder are the result of biceps abnormalities, cuff abnormalities, or both. This finding also complicates any study of the clinical utility of physical examination tests for biceps abnormality because the coexisting lesions can confound the test findings, decreasing the specificity.

Lastly, biceps tendon lesions are now known to include a wide range of abnormalities that can occur in many anatomic portions of the tendon. Taylor and colleagues[5] and Moon and colleagues[6] have divided the biceps tendon into 3 zones: an intra-articular portion (zone A), a portion beneath the transverse ligament (zone B), and a portion between the transverse ligament and the upper end of the pectoralis major insertion (zone C). Moon and colleagues[6] found that in patients with a 50% biceps tear in zone A, the lesions continued distally to zone B in 78% and to zone C in 72%. The lesions associated with long head of the biceps tendon abnormality include synovitis, partial tears, loose bodies, osteophytes, longitudinal splits, and stenosis.[7] The ways in which increasing knowledge of these abnormalities and their locations affect the physical examination are unknown.

Another lesion of the long head of the biceps tendon that complicates physical examination is biceps tendon subluxation, which has been noted since the nineteenth century.[8] Most subluxations are associated with abnormalities of the subscapularis tendon[9] or disorders of the biceps pulley system.[10] Biceps subluxations have been reported to be primarily movement of the tendon outside the groove lateral to the bicipital groove itself,[11] but most tendon subluxations are actually medial to the bicipital groove.[8,12] It is unknown to what degree a long head of the biceps tendon must be subluxated medially to create symptoms.

Similarly, lesions of the superior attachment of the long head of the biceps tendon to the superior labrum and supraglenoid tubercle (ie, superior labrum anterior and posterior [SLAP] lesions) make accurate diagnosis with a physical examination of the shoulder difficult. SLAP lesions have been classified into 13 variations.[13] The most common is type II, which is subdivided into 3 variants (anterior, posterior, and combined).[14] At least 17 physical examination tests have been described for SLAP lesions. Physical examination tests for SLAP lesions have the same limitations of studies of the long head of the biceps tendon lesions. It is uncommon for SLAP lesions to exist in isolation. Burkhart and colleagues[15] reported in their series of patients with type II SLAP lesions that 31% had partial rotator cuff tears. Kim and colleagues[16] found that 88% of patients with SLAP tears had coexisting abnormalities.

The complexity of biceps tendon lesions and how they produce symptoms is not well understood, and there is little consensus about which physical examination techniques are helpful in diagnosing these lesions. Most studies of biceps tendon abnormality involve patients with other lesions, but it may be that the combination of abnormalities contributes to pain and dysfunction. The goals of this article are to critically evaluate the effectiveness of the various physical examination tests for biceps tendon abnormalities and to discuss which tests are best for detecting biceps tendon abnormality.

EXAMINATION BASICS

When assessing patients for possible biceps tendon abnormalities, it is important to remember the value of a good history and the basics of shoulder examination. It is uncommon to have only a biceps tendon lesion in the differential diagnosis of shoulder pain or symptoms; as a result, it is important to obtain a complete medical history. For example, anterior shoulder pain in someone with a history of swelling in the arm could be caused by trauma or could suggest a contusion, fracture, tumor, or hematoma (for someone taking anticoagulants).

Because other lesions often coexist with biceps tendon abnormalities, it is important to consider various abnormalities when performing a shoulder examination. Patients should be undressed so that the examiner can see the musculature from the front and back and can compare sides (**Fig. 1**). A complete neurovascular examination is recommended, which includes strength testing of the rotator cuff muscles. Any paresthesia or weakness suggests that the cervical spine should be considered as a potential cause of the shoulder symptoms. Because subscapularis tendon abnormalities often coexist with biceps tendon abnormalities, testing of the subscapularis muscle and tendon should be performed. These tests include the lift-off test,[17] lift-off lag test,[18] resisted lift-off test,[17] and bear-hug test.[19] Previous literature has suggested that anterior shoulder instability can appear as a subluxating biceps tendon, so an anterior apprehension test or relocation test should be performed.[20] Suspected biceps tendon abnormality in overhead athletes should be evaluated with an

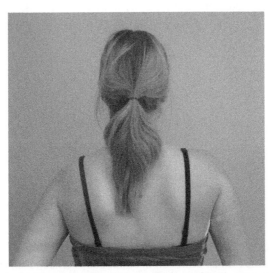

Fig. 1. Female patient with gown allowing visualization of both arms and shoulders.

examination of shoulder range of motion to detect glenohumeral internal rotation deficits,[15] neurologic deficits, or vascular lesions.

OBSERVATION

Patients with acute rupture of the biceps tendon typically have swelling and ecchymosis in the upper and middle regions of the brachium. After the swelling subsides, there is often a Popeye deformity, which is easy to visualize as a sagging biceps muscle belly resulting from the biceps tendon rupture. Atraumatic, painless swelling of the arm should be carefully examined for other possible explanations. If the swelling does not subside, it is important to ensure that the mass does not have characteristics of a tumor, such as firmness, overlying skin changes, or fixation to surrounding structures. The authors have experience with 2 masses in the arm that were originally diagnosed as biceps tendon ruptures but that proved to be malignant soft-tissue tumors.[21] In one case, the patient's arm was never examined by the surgeon, who relied on an erroneous MRI report; the second tumor was discovered because it was not in a typical location for a Popeye deformity.[21]

The Ludington Test

The Ludington test was first described in 1923 for the detection of complete tears of the biceps tendon.[22] As originally described, the patient placed the hands on the head with fingers intertwined and was directed to contract the arm muscles. The examiner then looked for asymmetry of the biceps muscles. The authors have found that the test can effectively be performed by having patients "show the biceps" by merely contracting the muscles with the elbows flexed (**Fig. 2**). Most full tears of the biceps tendon do not require this test to make the diagnosis. The Ludington test has some use after surgery when evaluating the tension on the biceps after tenodesis because it allows visual comparison with the other side (**Fig. 3**). The clinical utility of this test for other lesions of the biceps tendon has never been studied.

Biceps Tenderness

Biceps tenderness has been considered the hallmark of biceps tendon disorders, but there is little evidence supporting the validity or reliability of this. The biceps tendon runs in a groove covered by a fibrous extension of the subscapularis tendon

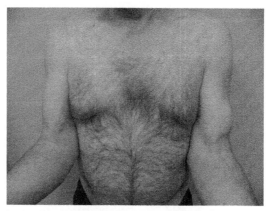

Fig. 2. In most patients with an acute full-thickness biceps tendon tear, the Popeye deformity is readily apparent on observation.

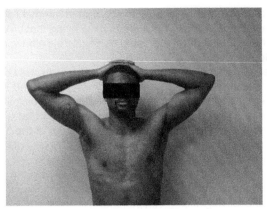

Fig. 3. The Ludington test is helpful for evaluating the asymmetry of the biceps muscles, especially after biceps tenodesis.

insertion.[23] The margins of the bicipital groove are marked by the lesser and greater tuberosities. These structures can be very difficult to palpate reliably, especially in individuals who have large deltoid muscles. Also, the anterior and superior quadrant of the shoulder has not only the insertion of the subscapularis and supraspinatus tendons but also the coracohumeral ligament, the conjoint tendon, and the biceps pulley system. It is difficult with palpation alone to determine which of these structures is contributing to pain.

The position of the arm when attempting to palpate the biceps tendon is recommended by Matsen and Kirby[24] to be 10° of internal rotation with the arm at the side (**Fig. 4**). With the arm in this position, the elbow is flexed and extended while the

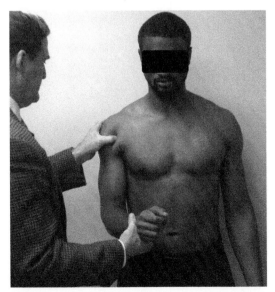

Fig. 4. Position for palpation of biceps tendon recommended by Matsen and Kirby.[24] The arm is at the side and in 10° of internal rotation.

examiner attempts to feel the tendon. With the arm in internal rotation, the biceps tendon is near the anterior joint line; the authors have found that by externally rotating the arm to 30° while concomitantly flexing and extending the elbow, the biceps tendon can be easier to locate (**Fig. 5**).[25]

There have been several anecdotal reports about the sensitivity of palpation of the biceps tendon for determining biceps abnormality. Crenshaw and Kilgore[26] reported that 88 of 89 patients who underwent biceps tenodesis had bicipital groove tenderness. An abstract by O'Brien and colleagues[27] suggested that biceps tenderness had a sensitivity of 98% and a specificity of 70% for lesions of the biceps labral complex. Only one published study[28] has examined the clinical utility of biceps tenderness for diagnosing partial biceps tendon tears, which were confirmed with arthroscopy. The investigators found that the sensitivity of biceps tenderness was 53%, the specificity was 54%, and the likelihood ratio was 1.13. They concluded that biceps tenderness was not reliable for diagnosing biceps tendon lesions.

BICEPS INSTABILITY TESTS

Instability of the biceps tendon can take several forms. One form is dynamic instability, in which the tendon subluxates out of the proximal bicipital groove anteriorly or posteriorly. The other form is a static subluxation typically seen in patients with lesions of the biceps pulley system with or without tears of the upper portion of the subscapularis tendon. The latter is much more common and can range from fixed subluxations at the bicipital groove to a completely displaced biceps tendon down to the level of the glenoid in the anterior compartment of the shoulder.

Testing for dynamic instability of the biceps tendon was described by Abbot and Saunders[29] in 1939. The test was performed by elevating the arm to full abduction and external rotation. The arm was then slowly brought down to the side while progressively internally rotating the shoulder. A positive test was a click or pop as

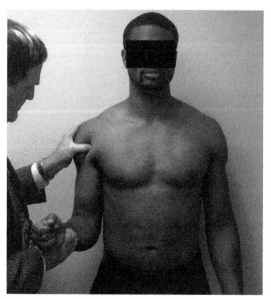

Fig. 5. If the arm is placed in 30° if external rotation, the biceps tendon is farther away from the anterior joint line and the two can be palpated separately.

the tendon slid into and out of the bicipital groove. Another approach is to elevate the arm 90° and internally and externally rotate the arm in an attempt to cause the tendon to slide in and out of the groove.

This test has never been studied in detail anatomically, biomechanically, or clinically. Dynamic biceps instability is much less common than it was thought to be during the first half of the twentieth century. In some instances, static subluxation of the biceps tendon was mistaken for a form of dynamic biceps instability. Typically, a biceps tendon that is subluxated over the superior edge of the lesser tuberosity medial to the bicipital groove does not cause clicking, catching, or locking. In their study of 71 patients with medially subluxated or dislocated biceps tendons, Walch and colleagues[9] reported no patients with clicking or jerking of the tendon on examination. Crepitus around the shoulder joint can also have various causes, and more evidence is required before these maneuvers can be recommended for making a diagnosis of biceps instability. In summary, dynamic biceps subluxations are extremely rare; the presence of a click or pain with circumduction of the shoulder should not be interpreted as biceps tendon instability or subluxation.

Yergason's Test

Yergason[30] reported the supination sign in 1931 as a test to detect "wear and tear of the long head of the biceps, or synovitis of its tendon sheath."[30(pp160)] The patient in this case report had full range of motion of the shoulder, tenderness at the greater tuberosity, and pain with active supination of the forearm. Yergason found that with the elbow flexed 90° at the side and the forearm pronated, resistance to active supination produced pain in the bicipital groove (**Fig. 6**).

Oddly, Yergason's test has been the subject of only 3 studies. The first was by Holtby and Razmjou[31] who studied 50 patients with partial or full tears of the biceps tendon. They found that the test had a sensitivity of 43%, specificity of 79%, overall accuracy of 63%, and likelihood ratio of 2.05. A second study by Parentis and colleagues[32] studied the usefulness of Yergason's test for diagnosing type II SLAP lesions. They reported a sensitivity of 93% but a specificity of only 13%. Both studies suggest that despite its popularity, Yergason's test does not accurately predict the

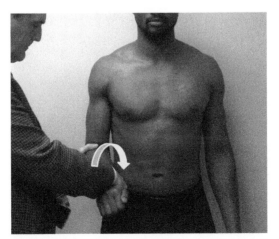

Fig. 6. Yergason's test is performed by having the patient fully pronate the forearm with the elbow bent 90°. The examiner then resists supination of the forearm by the patient. A positive test is anterior shoulder pain.

presence of biceps abnormality. Oh and colleagues[33] studied Yergason's test in patients proven arthroscopically to have type II SLAP lesions, reporting a sensitivity of 12% and specificity of 87%. In the authors' experience, a positive test is rare for any biceps tendon pathologies, and they no longer use this test when examining the shoulder.

Speed's Test

It is unknown when Speed's test was developed, but it was first attributed to Dr James Spencer Speed by Crenshaw and Kilgore[26] in 1966. According to their history, Dr Speed had pain in his shoulder when performing a straight leg test on patients with back pain. His pain occurred with his arm flexed in front of him, elbow extended, and forearm supinated (**Fig. 7**). This maneuver resulted in anterior shoulder pain, which was presumed to be caused by his biceps tendon.

Studies that have evaluated Speed's test are summarized in **Table 1**. Speed's test has been studied for its clinical utility for biceps lesions but also for SLAP lesions. In all 3 studies, the mean sensitivity was 57% (range, 32%–90%), specificity was 52% (range, 14%–78%), and overall accuracy was 61% (range, 56%–66%). One issue with Speed's test is that it can be positive in a variety of diagnoses. In the study by Gill and colleagues,[28] all patients with partial tears of the biceps tendon had other lesions, including rotator cuff tears, instability, rotator cuff syndrome with no cuff tears, and osteoarthritis. This study reiterates the difficulty of finding a cohort of patients with isolated biceps tendon lesions to determine the clinical utility of the tests for only biceps abnormality.

Lift-off Test

The lift-off test was first described by Gerber and Krushell[17] to detect subscapularis tendon tears. The association of subscapularis tendon tears with partial or full tears of the subscapularis tendon has been noted in several studies.[9,28] The lift-off test is performed by having patients place the hand up the lower back with the palm facing outward. Patients are then asked to lift the hand off the lower back. The test is positive if patients cannot lift the hand off the back.

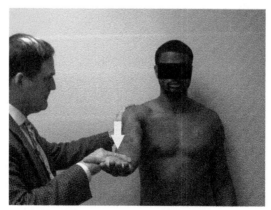

Fig. 7. Speed's test is performed with the arm forward flexed 90° with the elbow fully extended and the arm horizontally extended 10°. The patient resists downward force by the examiner, and a positive test is pain in the anterior shoulder.

Table 1
Diagnostic value of Speed's test for biceps tendon disorders in 3 studies

Study	Specificity (%)	Sensitivity (%)	NPV (%)	PPV (%)	Accuracy (%)
Bennett[51]	14	90	83	23	NR
Gill et al[28]	67	50	96	8	66
Holtby and Razmjou[52]	75	32	58	50	56

Abbreviations: NPV, negative predictive value; NR, not reported; PPV, positive predictive value.

In their study of partial tears of the biceps tendon, Gill and colleagues[28] found that a positive lift-off test had a sensitivity of 28% and a specificity of 89% for partial tears of the biceps. They concluded that the positive lift-off test could be explained by the association of partial biceps tears with partial tears of the subscapularis. Walch and colleagues[9] found that 71 of 445 (16%) rotator cuff tears had a subluxation or dislocation of the biceps tendon out of the bicipital groove at the time of surgery; however, all biceps subluxations or dislocations were associated with rotator cuff tears. They were unable to study the lift-off test in their cohort because some patients had too much pain with internal rotation up the back. They did find that all patients with biceps subluxation or dislocation had subscapularis tendon tears. Therefore, patients with subscapularis tendon tears have a high likelihood of having biceps tendon abnormality, and the treating surgeon should be aware of this association if surgery is being considered.

Biceps Entrapment Test

The biceps entrapment test was described by Boileau and colleagues[34] for diagnosing biceps entrapment. In this condition, the biceps tendon has a bulbous swelling just outside the joint in the bicipital groove (**Fig. 8**). This swelling acts like a trigger finger in that the bulbous area prevents full shoulder elevation without pain. The hallmark of biceps entrapment is the inability of the arm to reach full elevation. This

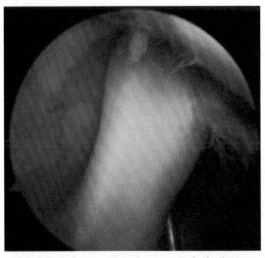

Fig. 8. Arthroscopic photograph from a posterior portal of a bulbous swelling of the biceps tendon, which can lead to biceps entrapment.

condition has been the subject of only one study, by Boileau and colleagues.[34] All of their 21 patients had a loss of full elevation (actively and passively) of 10° to 20°. All patients had anterior shoulder pain, which radiated into the neck in 8 patients and toward the elbow in 10 patients. Fifteen patients had tenderness over the bicipital groove, 10 had a positive Speed's test, and 17 had a positive Jobe's test. However, the definitive diagnosis in these patients could be made only at the time of surgery with an intraoperative test in which the hypertrophic portion of the tendon could be disengaged.[34]

SUPERIOR LABRUM ANTERIOR AND POSTERIOR LESIONS

The examination of the shoulder for SLAP lesions continues to be difficult despite the many available tests. Many studies have been hampered by poor design and the dispute over what is or is not a SLAP lesion. Arthroscopy is considered the gold standard for making the diagnosis, but reliability studies show that, although intraobserver reproducibility is generally good, interobserver reliability is poor. A study by Gobezie and colleagues[35] found that members of the American Orthopedic Society for Sports Medicine had poor agreement on grading when shown videos of SLAP lesions. Another study of more experienced surgeons who performed shoulder surgery frequently[36] reported intraobserver reliability of up to 86% but interobserver reliability only up to 65%. Many studies of SLAP lesions use modalities other than arthroscopy, such as MRI, magnetic resonance arthrography, or ultrasonography, as the gold standard for making the diagnosis.[37–39] Although it is beyond the scope of this review to evaluate the accuracy of those modalities, there remain questions about their accuracy and reliability, which can further confound results when comparing published studies.

The other issue with many studies of the examination for SLAP lesions is that they include not only SLAP lesions but also labral lesions at various locations in the joint. For example, Berg and Ciullo[40] reported high sensitivity of the SLAPprehension test for labral tears that were accompanied by a history of a click. However, the authors included Bankart lesions and SLAP lesions in their definition of a labral tear. Similarly, a study by Walsworth and colleagues[41] reported that if a patient had a history of a click and a positive anterior slide test, then the likelihood ratio for labral tears was infinity. Their study population included patients with SLAP tears and Bankart tears, which have completely different clinical presentations.

The third issue with many studies of the examination of SLAP lesions is that because isolated SLAP lesions are uncommon, many studies include coexisting lesions. For example, partial rotator cuff tears are common in overhead athletes who have SLAP lesions. Although SLAP repair provides pain relief for many patients, the high failure rate of SLAP repairs in athletes returning to a high level of play may be the result of rotator cuff tears and not SLAP lesions. Currently, no physical examination test distinguishes SLAP lesion pain from rotator cuff pain because they can both cause pain into the anterior or lateral shoulder.

There have been numerous studies of the clinical utility of physical examination tests for SLAP tears reported in a variety of sources.[16,25,42–45] However, 2 tests for the examination of SLAP tears deserve further analysis, provided later. The influence of combining tests to increase clinical utility is also summarized later.

Dynamic Shear Test

The dynamic shear test was first described by Cheung and O'Driscoll[46] at an American Academy of Orthopedic Surgeons meeting in 2007. The full description was not published until 2009.[47] This test is performed similarly to an anterior apprehension test, with the examiner behind patients holding the arm in abduction and external rotation (**Fig. 9**). The examiner then applies an anterior force on the shoulder as the arm is raised from approximately 70° of elevation to 120° of elevation and then down again. Pain in the posterior and superior shoulder indicates a positive test.[47]

Ben Kibler and colleagues[47] subsequently studied this test and reported a sensitivity of 72%, a specificity of 98%, and an extremely high likelihood ratio of 32 (**Table 2**). These findings suggested that it was highly diagnostic for SLAP lesions. The investigators used MRI and arthroscopy to make a definitive diagnosis.

The second published study of the dynamic shear test was less enthusiastic about its clinical utility. Cook and colleagues[42] studied the test in 86 patients and found that the sensitivity was 92%, the specificity was 20%, and the likelihood ratio was only 1.4. The gold standard in this study was diagnostic arthroscopy in all patients. The investigators concluded that the test was not useful for making the diagnosis of SLAP tears. However, it was subsequently pointed out by Ben Kibler and colleagues[47] that the test was not performed as described by Cheung and O'Driscoll[46] because the examination was performed with the examiner in front of the patients, making it difficult to direct an anterior force vector on the proximal humerus.

A third study of the dynamic shear test produced results lying between those of the two previously cited studies. Sodha and colleagues[48] performed the dynamic shear test in 674 patients who were undergoing diagnostic arthroscopy regardless of the diagnosis. Only 10 of these patients had an isolated SLAP lesion. The investigators found that, in patients with isolated SLAP lesions, the sensitivity of the dynamic shear test was 86%, the specificity was 52%, and the likelihood ratio was 3.6. However, there was another cohort of patients with a SLAP lesion who had other abnormalities, such as partial rotator cuff tears, full-thickness rotator cuff tears, shoulder instability, and acromioclavicular arthritis. In patients with concomitant lesions, the sensitivity was 58%, the specificity was 54%, and the odds ratio was 1.4. In other words, if a patient had an isolated SLAP lesion, the test was useful; but if there were other abnormalities, it was not as diagnostically accurate. Another issue with this test is that it is difficult to perform in some patients with anterior shoulder instability because it not only produces pain but can also produce profound apprehension that the shoulder might subluxate or dislocate. Further testing with more patients is necessary before this test can be recommended without reservation.

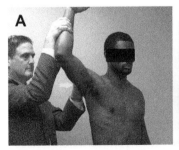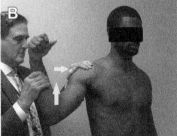

Fig. 9. The dynamic shear test is performed similarly to an anterior apprehension test with the examiner behind the patient and applying an anterior force to the shoulder as the arm is elevated from 70° to 120° (*A*) and back again (*B*). A positive test is posterior superior shoulder pain with or without a click.

Table 2
Diagnostic value of the dynamic shear test for labral tears in 3 different studies

Study	Specificity (%)	Sensitivity (%)	NPV (%)	PPV (%)	Likelihood Ratio	Accuracy (%)
Ben Kibler et al[47]	98	72	77	97	32	84
Cook et al[42]	30	89	60	69	1.3	NR
Sodha et al[53]	52	86	100	1.8	6.4	54

Abbreviations: NPV, negative predictive value; NR, not reported; PPV, positive predictive value.

Active Compression Test

The active compression test was described by O'Brien and colleagues[38] in 1998; it was reported that, for making the diagnosis of SLAP tears, the sensitivity was 100% and the specificity was 98.5%. The gold standard in this study was diagnostic arthroscopy. The active compression test is performed by asking patients to forward flex the arm 90°, horizontally adduct 10°, and internally rotate the arm so that the thumb points toward the floor (**Fig. 10**). The examiner then asks patients to resist a downward force on the arm. If there is a SLAP lesion, there should be a click or pain deep in the shoulder. Next, the examiner asks patients to keep the arm in the same position but to supinate the arm so that the palm faces the ceiling. The examiner then asks patients to resist a downward force on the arm. The test is considered positive if the pain stops or is diminished with the hand facing upward. The authors also indicated the test was helpful in diagnosing acromioclavicular joint problems, such as osteoarthritis and osteolysis.

This test was met with great enthusiasm and has become widely used and cited. However, there are several issues with the test. The first is that it requires patients to report where the pain is located, which is difficult for some patients, especially when the pain is deep in the shoulder as opposed to in the front or back of the shoulder. Some patients reported worse pain with the hand up as opposed to the hand down position, which was not part of the algorithm. Also, one study showed that a

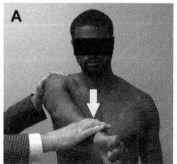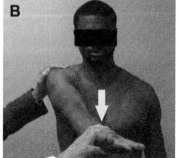

Fig. 10. The active compression test is performed with the arm forward flexed 90° and horizontally adducted 10°. It is performed first with the thumb down and the patient resisting a downward force by the examiner (*A*). The test is then performed with the palm up (*B*). A positive test is pain deep in the shoulder or a click with the palm down with less or no pain when the test is repeated with the palm up.

click in the shoulder is not a reliable sign of an SLAP lesion, with 5% of patients without SLAP lesions having a click.[44]

Subsequent studies of the active compression test of various populations produced different results (**Table 3**). A meta-analysis of the active compression test concluded that it was not diagnostic of SLAP lesions.[43] One study found that it had better clinical utility for diagnosing acromioclavicular disorders than SLAP lesions.[49] Despite these findings, this test remains popular, but its clinical utility is in question.

Multiple Physical Examination Tests for Superior Labrum Anterior and Posterior Lesions

Several studies have addressed the use of multiple tests to increase the likelihood of accurately diagnosing SLAP lesions.[33,41,44,47,50] One study used 3 physical examination tests: the compression rotation test, the anterior slide test, and the active compression test.[44] The accuracy of diagnosing SLAP tears was no higher with the use of all 3 tests in a given patient than with any one test or any combination of 2 tests.

Oh and colleagues[33] studied 26 patients with isolated type II SLAP tears and 42 patients with type II SLAP tears and other abnormalities. They examined all study group patients and 78 control group patients using 10 tests described for examining the shoulder (Speed's test, Yergason's test, anterior apprehension test, relocation test, compression rotation test, active compression test, anterior slide test, biceps load II test, Whipple test, and biceps groove tenderness). They did not find any one test to be sensitive and specific for a type II SLAP lesion. The sensitivities were highest for the Whipple (65%), apprehension (62%), and compression rotation (61%) tests, whereas the specificities were highest for the Yergason's (87%), biceps load II (78%), and active compression (53%) tests. The investigators found that combining 2 of the highly sensitive tests with one of the highly specific tests resulted in sensitivity of 70% and specificity of 95%. They also evaluated different combinations using an *and* function and an *or* function. If 2 tests from the highly sensitive group and one test from the highly specific group were chosen for evaluation, the sensitivity of the *or* combinations was approximately 75% and the specificity of the *and* combinations was approximately 90%.[33] The investigators concluded that no one test was pathognomonic for the diagnosis of SLAP lesions. Unfortunately, this schema never gained widespread use among clinicians because it was somewhat cumbersome and complex.

Table 3						
Diagnostic value of active compression test (O'Brien's test) for SLAP lesion/labral abnormality						
Study	Specificity (%)	Sensitivity (%)	NPV (%)	PPV (%)	Likelihood Ratio	Accuracy (%)
Ben Kibler et al[47]	61	38	31	67	0.96	53
Cook et al[42]	10	85	15	78	0.94	NR
Guanche and Jones[50]	73	63	87	40	NR	NR
Nakagawa et al[54]	60	54	52	62	NR	57
O'Brien et al[38]	98	100	94	100	NR	NR
Oh et al[33]	53	63	55	61	NR	NR
Parentis et al[55]	65	49	NR	NR	NR	NR
Stetson and Templin[39]	31	54	34	50	NR	NR

Abbreviations: NPV, negative predictive value; NR, not reported; PPV, positive predictive value.

SUMMARY

Currently, no single physical examination test can accurately diagnose biceps tendon abnormalities, including SLAP lesions. The location of the pain is not unique in biceps tendon abnormalities; in many instances, pain may be caused by other associated abnormalities. Pain in the anterior shoulder should perhaps be called *anterior shoulder pain syndrome* and not *biceps pain*. Similarly, the diagnosis of SLAP lesions through physical examination remains controversial, but it seems that the dynamic shear test can make the diagnosis more reliably than any other existing test. The authors currently consider pain in the overhead athlete deep in the shoulder or posterior-superior in the shoulder suspicious for a SLAP tear. The dynamic shear test has potential as a reliable test for making the diagnosis of SLAP tears, but it needs more study. Similarly, further study is needed to determine how to reliably and accurately diagnose biceps tendon conditions on physical examination without relying on diagnostic arthroscopy.

REFERENCES

1. Gerber C, Galantay RV, Hersche O. The pattern of pain produced by irritation of the acromioclavicular joint and the subacromial space. J Shoulder Elbow Surg 1998;7(4):352–5.
2. McFarland EG, Hobbs WR. The active shoulder: AC joint pain and injury. Your Patient and Fitness 1998;12(4):23–7.
3. Murthi AM, Vosburgh CL, Neviaser TJ. The incidence of pathologic changes of the long head of the biceps tendon. J Shoulder Elbow Surg 2000;9(5):382–5.
4. Chen CH, Hsu KY, Chen WJ, et al. Incidence and severity of biceps long head tendon lesion in patients with complete rotator cuff tears. J Trauma 2005;58(6): 1189–93.
5. Taylor SA, Khair MM, Gulotta LV, et al. Diagnostic glenohumeral arthroscopy fails to fully evaluate the biceps-labral complex. Arthroscopy 2015;31(2):215–24.
6. Moon SC, Cho NS, Rhee YG. Analysis of "hidden lesions" of the extra-articular biceps after subpectoral biceps tenodesis: the subpectoral portion as the optimal tenodesis site. Am J Sports Med 2015;43(1):63–8.
7. Hitchcock HH, Bechtol CO. Painful shoulder: observations of the role of the tendon of the long head of the biceps brachii in its causation. J Bone Joint Surg Am 1948;30(2):263–73.
8. Meyer AW. Spontaneous dislocation of the tendon of the long head of the biceps brachii. Arch Surg 1926;13(1):109–19.
9. Walch G, Nove-Josserand L, Boileau P, et al. Subluxations and dislocations of the tendon of the long head of the biceps. J Shoulder Elbow Surg 1998;7(2):100–8.
10. Braun S, Horan MP, Elser F, et al. Lesions of the biceps pulley. Am J Sports Med 2011;39(4):790–5.
11. Khazzam M, George MS, Churchill RS, et al. Disorders of the long head of biceps tendon. J Shoulder Elbow Surg 2012;21(1):136–45.
12. Meyer AW. Spontaneous dislocation and destruction of long head of biceps brachii. Fifty-nine instances. Arch Surg 1928;17:493–506.
13. Chang D, Mohana-Borges A, Borso M, et al. SLAP lesions: anatomy, clinical presentation, MR imaging diagnosis and characterization. Eur J Radiol 2008;68(1): 72–87.
14. Morgan CD, Burkhart SS, Palmeri M, et al. Type II SLAP lesions: three subtypes and their relationships to superior instability and rotator cuff tears. Arthroscopy 1998;14(6):553–65.

15. Burkhart SS, Morgan CD, Kibler WB. The disabled throwing shoulder: spectrum of pathology. Part I: pathoanatomy and biomechanics. Arthroscopy 2003;19(4): 404–20.

16. Kim TK, Queale WS, Cosgarea AJ, et al. Clinical features of the different types of SLAP lesions. An analysis of one hundred and thirty-nine cases. J Bone Joint Surg Am 2003;85(1):66–71.

17. Gerber C, Krushell RJ. Isolated rupture of the tendon of the subscapularis muscle. Clinical features in 16 cases. J Bone Joint Surg Br 1991;73(3):389–94.

18. Hertel R, Ballmer FT, Lambert SM, et al. Lag signs in the diagnosis of rotator cuff rupture. J Shoulder Elbow Surg 1996;5(4):307–13.

19. Barth JR, Burkhart SS, De Beer JF. The bear-hug test: a new and sensitive test for diagnosing a subscapularis tear. Arthroscopy 2006;22(10):1076–84.

20. Eakin CL, Faber KJ, Hawkins RJ, et al. Biceps tendon disorders in athletes. J Am Acad Orthop Surg 1999;7(5):300–10.

21. Tantisricharoenkul G, Tan EW, Fayad LM, et al. Malignant soft tissue tumors of the biceps muscle mistaken for proximal biceps tendon rupture. Orthopedics 2012; 35(10):e1548–52, 898.

22. Ludington NA. Rupture of the long head of the biceps flexor cubiti muscle. Ann Surg 1923;77(3):358–63.

23. Brasseur JL. The biceps tendons: from the top and from the bottom. J Ultrasound 2012;15(1):29–38.

24. Matsen FA III, Kirby RM. Office evaluation and management of shoulder pain. Orthop Clin North Am 1982;13(3):453–75.

25. McFarland EG. Examination of the biceps tendon and superior labrum anterior and posterior (SLAP) lesions. In: Kim TK, Park HB, El Rassi G, et al, editors. Examination of the shoulder: the complete guide. New York: Thieme; 2006. p. 213–43.

26. Crenshaw AH, Kilgore WE. Surgical treatment of bicipital tenosynovitis. J Bone Joint Surg Am 1966;48(8):1496–502.

27. O'Brien SJ, Newman AM, Taylor S, et al. The accurate diagnosis of biceps-labral complex lesions with MRI and "3-pack" physical examination: a retrospective analysis with prospective validation. Orthop J Sports Med 2013;1(Suppl 4).

28. Gill HS, El Rassi G, Bahk MS, et al. Physical examination for partial tears of the biceps tendon. Am J Sports Med 2007;35(8):1334–40.

29. Abbot LC, Saunders JB. Acute traumatic dislocation of the tendon of long head of biceps brachii. A report of six cases with operative findings. Surgery 1939;6(6): 817–40.

30. Yergason RM. Supination sign. J Bone Joint Surg Am 1931;13(1):160.

31. Holtby R, Razmjou H. Accuracy of the Speed's and Yergason's tests in detecting biceps pathology and SLAP lesions: comparison with arthroscopic findings. Arthroscopy 2004;20(3):231–6.

32. Parentis MA, Glousman RE, Mohr KS, et al. An evaluation of the provocative tests for superior labral anterior posterior lesions. Am J Sports Med 2006;34(2):265–8.

33. Oh JH, Kim JY, Kim WS, et al. The evaluation of various physical examinations for the diagnosis of type II superior labrum anterior and posterior lesion. Am J Sports Med 2008;36(2):353–9.

34. Boileau P, Ahrens PM, Hatzidakis AM. Entrapment of the long head of the biceps tendon: the hourglass biceps – a cause of pain and locking of the shoulder. J Shoulder Elbow Surg 2004;13(3):249–57.

35. Gobezie R, Zurakowski D, Lavery K, et al. Analysis of interobserver and intraobserver variability in the diagnosis and treatment of SLAP tears using the Snyder classification. Am J Sports Med 2008;36(7):1373–9.

36. Jia X, Yokota A, McCarty EC, et al. Reproducibility and reliability of the Snyder classification of superior labral anterior posterior lesions among shoulder surgeons. Am J Sports Med 2011;39(5):986–91.

37. Mimori K, Muneta T, Nakagawa T, et al. A new pain provocation test for superior labral tears of the shoulder. Am J Sports Med 1999;27(2):137–42.

38. O'Brien SJ, Pagnani MJ, Fealy S, et al. The active compression test: a new and effective test for diagnosing labral tears and acromioclavicular joint abnormality. Am J Sports Med 1998;26(5):610–3.

39. Stetson WB, Templin K. The crank test, the O'Brien test, and routine magnetic resonance imaging scans in the diagnosis of labral tears. Am J Sports Med 2002;30(6):806–9.

40. Berg EE, Ciullo JV. A clinical test for superior glenoid labral or 'SLAP' lesions. Clin J Sport Med 1998;8(2):121–3.

41. Walsworth MK, Doukas WC, Murphy KP, et al. Reliability and diagnostic accuracy of history and physical examination for diagnosing glenoid labral tears. Am J Sports Med 2008;36(1):162–8.

42. Cook C, Beaty S, Kissenberth MJ, et al. Diagnostic accuracy of five orthopedic clinical tests for diagnosis of superior labrum anterior posterior (SLAP) lesions. J Shoulder Elbow Surg 2012;21(1):13–22.

43. Hegedus EJ, Goode AP, Cook CE, et al. Which physical examination tests provide clinicians with the most value when examining the shoulder? Update of a systematic review with meta-analysis of individual tests. Br J Sports Med 2012; 46(14):964–78.

44. McFarland EG, Kim TK, Savino RM. Clinical assessment of three common tests for superior labral anterior-posterior lesions. Am J Sports Med 2002;30(6):810–5.

45. Meserve BB, Cleland JA, Boucher TR. A meta-analysis examining clinical test utility for assessing superior labral anterior posterior lesions. Am J Sports Med 2009; 37(11):2252–8.

46. Cheung EV, O'Driscoll SW. The dynamic labral shear test for superior labral anterior posterior tears of the shoulder. Podium presentation at the 76th Annual Meeting of the American Academy of Orthopaedic Surgeons. San Diego (CA), February 14–17, 2007.

47. Ben Kibler W, Sciascia AD, Hester P, et al. Clinical utility of traditional and new tests in the diagnosis of biceps tendon injuries and superior labrum anterior and posterior lesions in the shoulder. Am J Sports Med 2009;37(9):1840–7.

48. Sodha S, Joseph J, Borade A, et al. Clinical assessment of the dynamic shear test for SLAP lesions. Presented at The American College of Sports Medicine 62nd Annual Meeting. San Diego (CA), May 26–30, 2015.

49. Chronopoulos E, Kim TK, Park HB, et al. Diagnostic value of physical tests for isolated chronic acromioclavicular lesions. Am J Sports Med 2004;32(3):655–61.

50. Guanche CA, Jones DC. Clinical testing for tears of the glenoid labrum. Arthroscopy 2003;19(5):517–23.

51. Bennett WF. Specificity of the Speed's test: arthroscopic technique for evaluating the biceps tendon at the level of the bicipital groove. Arthroscopy 1998;14(8): 789–96.

52. Holtby R, Razmjou H. Impact of work-related compensation claims on surgical outcome of patients with rotator cuff related pathologies: a matched case-control study. J Shoulder Elbow Surg 2010;19(3):452–60.

53. Sodha S, Joseph J, Borade A, et al. Clinical assessment of the dynamic shear test for SLAP lesions. Presented at The American Orthopaedic Society for Sports Medicine (AOSSM) annual meeting. Orlando (FL), July 9–12, 2015.

54. Nakagawa S, Yoneda M, Hayashida K, et al. Forced shoulder abduction and elbow flexion test: a new simple clinical test to detect superior labral injury in the throwing shoulder. Arthroscopy 2005;21(11):1290–5.
55. Parentis MA, Mohr KJ, Elattrache NS. Disorders of the superior labrum: review and treatment guidelines. Clin Orthop Relat Res 2002;(400):77–87.

How Accurate Are We in Detecting Biceps Tendinopathy?

Ryan M. Carr, MD[a], Yousef Shishani, MD[b], Reuben Gobezie, MD[c],*

KEYWORDS

- Biceps tendinitis • Biceps tendinopathy • MRI • Histology • Anterior shoulder pain

KEY POINTS

- Although certain provocative maneuvers can help to guide the decision making process, they are nonspecific and imperfect.
- Biceps tendon pain may be more difficult to discern in the absence of a frank tear or changes in signal intensity as perceived by MRI.
- Studies using MRI or arthroscopy as the gold standard may miss this diagnosis.

INTRODUCTION: NATURE OF THE PROBLEM

Anterior shoulder pain can result from several different pathologies, including rotator cuff tears, rotator cuff tendinitis, subacromial bursitis, impingement (subacromial and subcoracoid), acromioclavicular joint arthritis, and anterior labral tears, as well as biceps tendinopathy, instability, and tendon tears. Advanced imaging studies including MRI can help to delineate many of these pathologies with the exception of the biceps tendon, which is frequently missed or misdiagnosed. A strong clinical suspicion may be the most important diagnostic parameter based on patient history and clinical examination findings. However, direct visualization during arthroscopy may be the most sensitive and specific diagnostic modality.

INDICATIONS FOR IMAGING OF THE BICEPS

What Do We Know About Biceps Tendinopathy?

In the author's experience, the clinical symptoms of biceps tendinopathy are anterior shoulder pain or pain down "the side of the arm" that occurs with rotation of the

R. Gobezie receives royalties from Arthrex Inc.

[a] Cleveland Akron Shoulder & Elbow Fellowship (CASE), Cleveland Shoulder Institute, University Hospitals of Cleveland, 3999 Richmond Road, Beachwood, OH 44122, USA; [b] Cleveland Shoulder Institute, University Hospitals of Cleveland, 3999 Richmond Road, Beachwood, OH 44122, USA; [c] Cleveland Akron Shoulder & Elbow Fellowship (CASE), Cleveland Shoulder Institute, University Hospitals of Cleveland, 3999 Richmond Road, Beachwood, OH 44122, USA
* Corresponding author.
E-mail address: reuben.gobezie@uhhospitals.org

shoulder, such as when patients reach in the backseat of their car, tuck in their pants in, or fasten their bra. The patients often have pain at night that wakes them from sleep, especially if they are side sleepers (which often requires external rotation and adduction). The bicipital groove is tender on palpation and many, but not all, of these patients have a positive Speed's and/or O'Brien's test. In the author's experience, physical therapy is not often helpful. Activity modification in the form of avoidance of rotation with resistance such as abduction dumbbells, fly-press exercises, serving a tennis ball, or throwing a baseball can improve symptoms (if they are not too restrictive to be tolerated by the patient). If 3 to 4 weeks of activity modification does not resolve the patient's symptoms, the author recommends use of an ultrasound-guided corticosteroid injection into the bicipital groove as both a diagnostic and potentially therapeutic intervention.

Biceps tendon pain has recently been characterized by histologic analysis. Streit and colleagues[1] analyzed 26 patients after a subpectoral biceps tenodesis for anterior shoulder pain located along the biceps groove. Clinical indication of biceps tendinopathy was made based on the physical examination, including increased pain owing to direct biceps groove palpation, Speed's test, and the O'Brien test.[1] Traditionally, the clinical suspicion of biceps tendinopathy may be an indication for acquisition of an MRI to evaluate for the presence of a biceps tear. In the study by Streit and colleagues,[1] a standard noncontrast MRI study was performed before proceeding with surgery. More important, histologic analysis was performed on all patients to determine if biceps pain truly results from inflammation. At the time of the index procedure, Streit and colleagues[1] excised a portion of the long head of the biceps tendon and sheath of tenosynovium located 2 cm proximal to the musculotendinous junction and sent the sample for histologic analysis. Analysis was performed by a single pathologist with extensive experience in evaluating musculoskeletal tissue.[1] The biceps tendon was evaluated for changes in tenocyte morphology, ground substance, vascularity, and organization of the collagen bundles using the modified Bonar score.[1] The synovial sheath was also evaluated looking at hypercellularity, and vascularity and was graded on the percent of involvement.[1]

Before operative intervention, 100% of patients demonstrated pain along the biceps groove, and 93.3% demonstrated both a positive Speed and O'Brien test, the usual clinical indications for biceps tendinitis.[1] Arthroscopic evaluation demonstrated a superior labral anterior–posterior (SLAP) tear in 86.7%, and a biceps tendon tear distal to the root in 33.3%.[1] Histologic analysis found that all of the specimens demonstrated changes in tenocyte size (**Fig. 1**), ground substance morphology (**Fig. 2**), collagen bundle organization (**Figs. 3** and **4**), and vascularity (**Fig. 5**).[1] Similarly, 93% of the specimens demonstrated grade 2 or 3 changes as determined by the modified Bonar scale for tenocyte morphology.[1] Out of all 26 specimens, 96% demonstrated grade 2 changes in ground substance morphology.[1] Changes in vascularity were noted in all specimens with 58.6% demonstrating at least grade 2 changes.[1] All specimens demonstrated fibrosis and myxoid degeneration.[1] Two specimens demonstrated mild chronic inflammatory changes with the remaining samples demonstrating degenerative changes in the absence of any inflammatory process.[1] The synovial sheath demonstrated proliferation of the synovial cell in the absence of inflammation (**Fig. 6**).[1]

These changes indicate that biceps pain and clinical evaluation are indicative of biceps tendinopathy, not tendinitis, consistent with other tendinopathies seen throughout the body. Studies evaluating these changes indicate they are linked to an alteration in the signaling pathway for cytokines and growth hormones in response to stress and mechanical loads perceived by the tendon.[2,3] Additional studies evaluating this phenomenon have resulted in similar conclusions.[4]

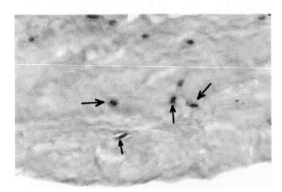

Fig. 1. Increased tenocyte cell size and nucleus (*arrows*).

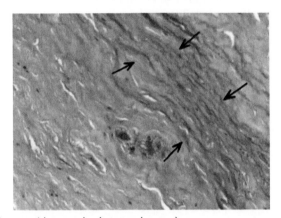

Fig. 2. Increase in myxoid ground substance (*arrows*).

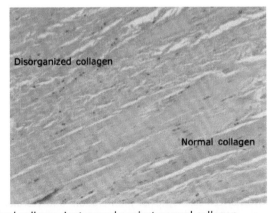

Fig. 3. Disorganized collagen juxtaposed against normal collagen.

Fig. 4. Fragmented collagen (*asterisk*) as seen on polarized light microscopy. Normal collagen (*double asterisk*).

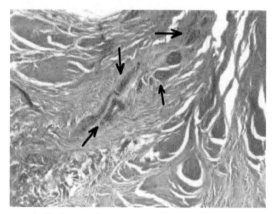

Fig. 5. Increase in vascularity (*arrows*).

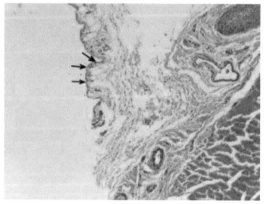

Fig. 6. Increase in synovial cell size, synovial proliferation, and vascularity of the biceps tenosynovium (*arrows*).

Indications for Imaging

The studies evaluating the imaging of biceps pathology using MRI scans have failed to show high sensitivity and/or specificity for identifying tears or tendinopathy. Many of these studies were performed using lower resolution MRI scanners with magnets that have less than 3 T. In the author's opinion, the absence of biceps pathology on MRI imaging does not necessarily exclude the presence of tendinopathy.

STUDIES EVALUATING THE EFFICACY OF MRI

In addition to clinical evaluation, imaging studies including noncontrast MRI have been evaluated as a diagnostic modality for biceps pathology. Dubrow and colleagues[5] evaluated the efficacy of noncontrast MRI in detecting biceps tendinopathy in conjunction with diagnostic arthroscopy. Sixty-six patients suspected of having biceps tendinopathy, partial or complete biceps tendon tears, biceps instability, or SLAP tear were evaluated using noncontrast MRI.[5] All patients had previously failed conservative measures, including physical therapy, activity modification, and corticosteroid injections for a period exceeding 4 months.[5] Patients with a prior history of shoulder surgery, fracture, inflammatory arthritis, or adhesive capsulitis were excluded.[5] MRI was evaluated by a single fellowship-trained musculoskeletal radiologist.[5]

The biceps tendon was evaluated for complete and partial tears including intraarticular splits or fraying, as well as intact tendons demonstrating degenerative changes (Fig. 7).[5] These findings were compared with arthroscopic evaluation looking at inflammation as well as longitudinal, partial, and complete tears of the biceps tendon and pulley.[5] Average time between MRI and arthroscopy was 1.55 months.[5] Sensitivity, specificity, negative predictive value (NPV), and positive predictive value (PPV) were calculated for the normal, partial, and complete biceps tendon tears (Fig. 8) and was found to be poor in detecting biceps tendon pathology in comparison to arthroscopy.[5] The concordance rate between MRI and arthroscopy was also evaluated, with equivalent findings being detected only 34.9% of the time.[5] Additional studies have also evaluated MRI imaging in detecting biceps pathology with similar findings.[6]

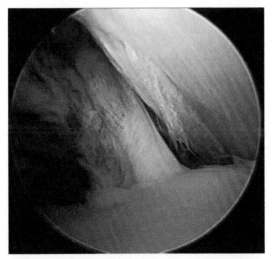

Fig. 7. Tear involving the long head of the biceps and partial tear in the biceps pulley.

MRI:

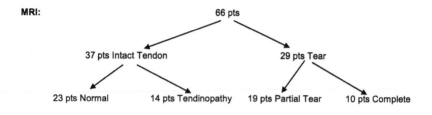

Arthroscopy:

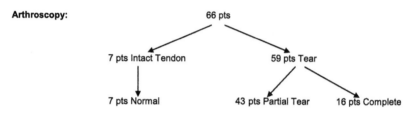

MRI Evaluation of Anterior Shoulder Pain				
	Sensitivity	Specificity	PPV	NPV
Normal LHB Tendon	85.7%	70.0%	25.0%	97.7%
Partial LHB Tear	27.7%	84.2%	81.2%	32.0%
Complete LHB Tear	56.3%	98.0%	90.0%	87.5%

Fig. 8. Detecting biceps tendinopathy: Noncontrast MRI in conjunction with diagnostic arthroscopy. LHB, long head of biceps; NPV, negative predictive value; PPV, positive predictive value; pts, patients.

A similar study was conducted comparing the accuracy in detecting biceps tendon pathology in patients with a rotator cuff tear with and without biceps tendon pathology using a 1.5-T MRI.[7] These findings were compared with arthroscopy at the time of the index procedure for rotator cuff repair.[7] This prospective study evaluated 183 patients with an interval between MRI and surgery of 179 days.[7] The percentage of agreement between the imaging study and the time to surgery was not significant, indicating that the lapse in time did impact the accuracy of the evaluation.[7]

Each patient was evaluated for biceps tendinopathy, and partial and complete tears.[7] In this sample population, no patient had isolated biceps tendinopathy owing to the presence of a rotator cuff tear.[7] Therefore, all patients had at least a partial or complete biceps tendon tear for this evaluation. Additional studies have noted a pathologic change in the biceps tendon in association with rotator cuff tears, which seems to correspond with the results from this study.[8,9] MRI demonstrated a 0.27 and 0.86 sensitivity and specificity for partial biceps tendon tears, respectively, indicating that MRI is not very reliable in detecting partial biceps tendon tears.[7] Seventy-three percent of partial biceps tendon tears were missed and 14% of normal biceps tendons were misdiagnosed as partial biceps tendon tears (**Fig. 9**).[7] In patients with full-thickness biceps tendon tears, 54% were correctly identified, leaving 46% incorrectly identified.[7] MRI was therefore much better at detecting intact biceps tendons, which occurred 98% of the time.[7] The study concluded that MRI has a high specificity for detecting complete rupture, but was unreliable in detecting partial tears.[7]

Ultrasonography has also been used to evaluate biceps tendon pathology. In comparison with arthroscopy, ultrasonography demonstrates reliability in detecting full-thickness biceps tendon tears, biceps tendon subluxation, and dislocation. However,

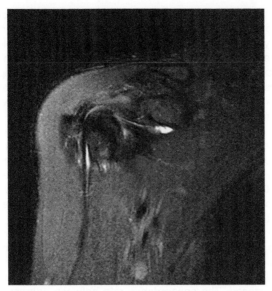

Fig. 9. T2 MRI of the same patient and normal biceps pathology as reported by radiology.

ultrasonography has a low sensitivity (49%) in detecting partial biceps tendon tears and, therefore, like MRI, is not reliable in this regard.[10]

Studies Considering the Speed and Yergason Tests

Various studies have evaluated the effectiveness of the Speed and Yergason tests in evaluating proximal biceps tendon pathology. These studies used both MRI and arthroscopy as the gold standard in which to compare these findings.[11,12] In a study by Calis and colleagues,[11] the authors compared the Speed and Yergason test results with that of MRI, using increased signal intensity, thinning or irregularity, or disruption of the tendon as an indication of biceps pathology. In this study, they found both a low sensitivity and specificity for the Speed test (68.5% and 55.5%, respectively) and the Yergason test (37.0% and 86.1%, respectively).[11] Bennett[12] evaluated the effectiveness of the Speed test against arthroscopic evaluation of the biceps tendon using inflammation, tearing, avulsion, or SLAP lesion as the endpoint. He found a sensitivity of 90%, specificity of 13.8%, PPV 23%, and NPV 83%.[12] He concluded that the Speed test is sensitive for macroscopic biceps pathology.[12]

Another study evaluating the effectiveness of the Speed and Yergason tests versus that of arthroscopy concluded that physical examination findings are inconsistent and are unlikely to change pretest diagnosis (Speed test: sensitivity 32%, specificity 75%, PPV 50%, NPV 58%) (Yergason test: sensitivity 43%, specificity 79%, PPV 60%, NPV 65%).[13] They did note that their analysis differed from that of other previously reported studies, and that this variability may be owing to inherent weaknesses in study design for all studies.[13]

DISCUSSION

Although certain provocative maneuvers can help guide our decision making process, they are nonspecific and imperfect. Furthermore, biceps tendon pain as it relates to tendinopathy may be more difficult to discern in the absence of a frank tear or changes in signal intensity as perceived by magnetic resonance imaging. Studies that use MRI or arthroscopy as the gold standard may therefore miss this diagnosis.

Histologic analysis of the biceps tendon demonstrates microscopic changes in the architecture of the biceps tendon in patients with biceps tendon pain. These changes may not be perceived by the naked eye or by advanced imaging studies in the absence of gross pathologic changes. The previous notion or terminology, which described biceps "tendinitis," implies inflammatory pathology. However, histologic analysis actually reveals the absence of inflammatory cells. Instead, we see changes in tenocyte size, collagen organization, ground substance, and vascularity. This is more accurately termed "tendinopathy" and may relate to signal changes in cytokines and growth hormones owing to a perceived change in stress and altered mechanics of the tendon. Patients may, therefore, exhibit symptoms in the absence of a biceps tendon tear. Furthermore, changes that we typically associate with inflammation should also be absent. Therefore, making the diagnosis of biceps tendinopathy may be more difficult than originally perceived.

Historically, we have used changes in signal sequence as seen on magnetic resonance imaging to indicate pathologic change. However, studies that have evaluated the effectiveness of MRI indicate that this study is more accurate in detecting complete biceps tendon tears.[5] Incomplete tears or tendinopathy are more likely to be missed or misdiagnosed. The concordance rate between arthroscopy and MRI for biceps tendon pathology remains low, indicating that MRI is imperfect at detecting this pathology.

Biceps tendon pain can result from biceps tendon tears, as well as from biceps tendinopathy, with those originating from tendinopathy more difficult to discern. Therefore, one must have a strong clinical suspicion based on patient history, and physical examination findings. At our institution, we do not rely on MRI to evaluate the biceps tendon, instead using it as an adjunct to help identify other shoulder pathology.

SUMMARY

Biceps tendon pain in the absence of biceps tendon tears is associated with microscopic changes consistent with tendinopathy. In the author's opinion, biceps tendon pain is best recognized by utilizing a combination of clinical symptoms of pain with rotation, physical examination with tenderness over the bicipital groove and, finally, ultrasound-guided injection into the bicipital groove to confirm the diagnosis. Tendinopathy is often missed by MRI.

REFERENCES

1. Streit JJ, Shishani Y, Rodgers M, et al. Tendinopathy of the long head of the biceps tendon: histopathologic analysis of the extra-articular biceps tendon and tenosynovium. Open Access J Sports Med 2015;6:63–70.
2. Zhange J, Wang JH. Mechanobiological rezones of tendon stem cells: implications of tendon homeostasis and pathogenesis of tendinopathy. J Orthop Res 2010;28(5):639–43.
3. Bi Y, Ehirchiou D, Kilts TM, et al. Identification of tendon stem/progenitor cells and the role of the extracellular matrix in their niche. Nat Med 2007;13(10):1219–27.
4. Longo UG, Franceschi F, Ruzzini L, et al. Characteristics at haematoxylin and eosin staining of ruptures of the long head of the biceps tendon. Br J Sports Med 2009;43(8):603–7.

5. Dubrow SJ, Streit JJ, Shishani Y, et al. Diagnostic accuracy in detecting tears in the proximal biceps tendon using standard nonenhancing shoulder MRI. Open Access J Sports Med 2014;5:81–7.
6. Mohtadi NG, Vellet AD, Clark ML, et al. A prospective, double-blind comparison of magnetic resonance imaging and arthroscopy in the evaluation of patients presenting with shoulder pain. J Shoulder Elbow Surg 2004;13(3):258–65.
7. Razmjou H, Fournier-Gosselin S, Christakis M, et al. Accuracy of magnetic resonance imaging in detecting biceps pathology in patients with rotator cuff disorders: comparison with arthroscopy. J Shoulder Elbow Surg 2015. [Epub ahead of print].
8. Harrison AK, Flatow EL. Subacromial impingement syndrome. J Am Acad Orthop Surg 2011;19(11):701–8.
9. Murthi AM, Vosburgh CL, Neviaser TJ. The incidence of pathologic changes of the long head of the biceps tendon. J Shoulder Elbow Surg 2000;9(5):382–5.
10. Armstrong A, Teefey SA, Wu T, et al. The efficacy of ultrasound in the diagnosis of long head of the biceps tendon pathology. J Shoulder Elbow Surg 2006;15(1): 7–11.
11. Calis M, Akgun K, Birtaine M, et al. Diagnostic values of clinical diagnostic tests in subacromial impingement syndrome. Ann Rheum Dis 2000;59:44–7.
12. Bennett WF. Specificity of the speed's test: arthroscopic technique for evaluating the biceps tendon at the level of the bicipital groove. Arthroscopy 1998;8:789–96.
13. Holtby R, Razmjou H. Accuracy of the Speed's and Yergason's tests in detecting biceps pathology and slap lesions: comparison with arthroscopic findings. Arthroscopy 2004;20(3):231–6.

Nonoperative Management (Including Ultrasound-Guided Injections) of Proximal Biceps Disorders

Mark Schickendantz, MD*, Dominic King, DO

KEYWORDS

- Long head of biceps tendon • Inflammation • Instability • Rupture
- Ultrasound guidance

KEY POINTS

- Diagnosis and nonoperative management of long head of biceps tendon disorders are categorized as inflammation, instability and rupture.
- Specific protocols that address these categories are necessary for comprehensive treatment.
- Musculoskeletal ultrasound scan can provide real-time imaging of long head of biceps tendon and associated structure conditions and can provide guidance for increased accuracy of injection.
- A multiphase physical rehabilitation program allows for progressive increase in muscle strength while possibly providing protection against further long head of biceps tendon and associated structure injury.
- Regenerative injection therapies may provide significant benefit in the healing and rehabilitation process of LHBT and associated structure conditions; however, further research is needed to define protocols and patient populations likely to benefit from this therapy.

LONG HEAD OF BICEPS TENDON

Long head of biceps tendon (LHBT) disorders are commonly encountered issues in a sports medicine practice; however, because of the complexity of this structure, the exact diagnosis can be challenging to make, and management can be controversial. LHBT disorders can present as isolated conditions, but they are commonly associated with additional shoulder issues, such as rotator cuff tears, in up to 90% of cases.[1,2]

The authors have no commercial or financial conflicts of interest or funding sources.
All figures and illustrations are original work by D. King, DO.
Cleveland Clinic Center for Sports Health, 5555 Transportation Boulevard, Garfield Heights, OH 44125, USA
* Corresponding author.
E-mail address: schickm@ccf.org

Clin Sports Med 35 (2016) 57–73
http://dx.doi.org/10.1016/j.csm.2015.08.006
0278-5919/16/$ – see front matter © 2016 Elsevier Inc. All rights reserved.

Patients with LHBT conditions commonly present with either pain, weakness, or a sense of instability.[2] An understanding of the normal anatomy and varied disorders of this complex area of the shoulder is crucial to present an efficacious nonsurgical management strategy.

Anatomy

The anatomy of the LHBT and associated structures is elegantly complex (**Box 1**).[1–9] The LHBT, specifically at the level of the rotator cuff interval, is held in place and supported by several different anatomic structures (**Fig. 1**).[1,3,4,6,7]

Pathologic Conditions

The 3 main categories of LHBT disorders are inflammation, instability and rupture. Multiple examples of these conditions are encountered when evaluating a patient with suspected LHBT injury (**Box 2**).[3,4,7] Inflammation can cause weakening and eventual damage to the stabilizing structures of the LHBT, leading to instability. Instability can cause improper LHBT mechanics and abnormal stresses on the LHBT and associated structures, predisposing to inflammation of the LHBT. Chronic inflammation and instability can predispose the LHBT to partial or complete rupture (**Fig. 2**).[1,2,4,6,7] This spectrum of disorders is most commonly seen at the level of the rotator interval (**Fig. 3**).[1,3,4,6,7]

PATIENT EVALUATION
Clinical Presentation/Physical Examination

Patients with biceps disorders commonly present with either pain, weakness, or a sense of instability.[2] To accurately delineate these symptoms and arrive at a comprehensive functional diagnosis, an appropriate history and physical examination need to

---

Box 1
Anatomic features of the LHBT

Origin

- Superior glenoid labrum and supraglenoid tubercle

Length

- 9 to 10 cm

Arterial Supply to Biceps

- Anterior circumflex humeral artery (major)
- Suprascapular artery (minor)

Innervation

- Branches of the musculocutaneous nerve (C5)

Additional information

- The LHBT is intra-articular and extrasynovial.
- The tendon exits the glenohumeral joint at a 30° to 40° angle via the biceps reflection pulley and bicipital groove.
- As the tendon exits the glenohumeral joint, it passes underneath the coracohumeral ligament and through the rotator interval.
- There is a watershed region located between the reflection pulley and bicipital groove.
- The proximal one-third of the tendon has the highest degree of sensory innervation.

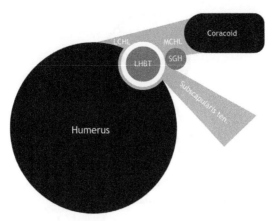

Fig. 1. Normal anatomic diagram of the LHBT sheath and associated structures. LCHL, lateral coracohumeral ligament; MCHL, medial coracohumeral ligament; SGH, superior glenohumeral ligament.

be completed. The history should contain elements specific to a patient presenting with anterior shoulder pain but should also note associated symptoms of additional local conditions (**Table 1**).[3,4,7,10,11] With regard to the physical examination, several provocative tests can be performed to elicit pain, weakness, or instability of the LHBT. These tests have varying degrees of sensitivity and specificity, and it is important to remember that other shoulder conditions may present similarly, which makes a diagnosis of LHBT disorders difficult by physical examination alone.[12] However, when incorporating the patient history, clinical presentation, and a targeted, specific physical examination, the examiner can begin to generate a narrowed differential diagnosis.[10]

When evaluating the LHBT, there are 3 main physical examination findings to note.[10] First, observe for symmetry: observe for symmetric contour of the biceps with the patient flexing at 90° of shoulder abduction, looking for a peaked prominence of the biceps

---

Box 2
Overview of LHBT disorders

Inflammation

- Primary tendinitis: Overuse, inflammation in the bicipital groove without associated shoulder pathology

- Secondary tendinitis: chronic inflammation with associated shoulder pathology, bicep tendinosis, rotator cuff fatigue, loss of humeral head containment, increased subacromial contact forces, instability

Instability

- Subluxation or dislocation of the LHBT from the bicipital groove secondary to rotator interval injury, injury to medial sling (coracohumeral ligament/superior glenohumeral ligament), tearing of lateral coracohumeral ligament, supraspinatus and subscapularis tendon injuries, SLAP injuries (IV/V/VI)

Rupture

- Partial split tearing, fraying or complete rupture secondary to overuse, attrition, impingement, chronic inflammation/instability

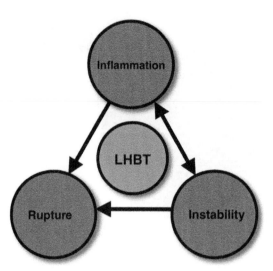

Fig. 2. LHBT pathologic condition overview.

muscle compared with the contralateral side, indicating rupture. The Speed's test is performed by resisting shoulder forward flexion with the patient's arm supinated, eliciting anterior shoulder pain at the LHBT, indicating inflammation. Finally, the Yergason's test is performed by resisting supination with the patient's arm at the side of the body and elbow in 90° of flexion, eliciting anterior shoulder pain at the LHBT with or without palpable subluxation of the LHBT, indicating inflammation and/or instability.[10]

Differential Diagnosis

The shoulder complex contains many bony landmarks that can be palpated through the skin. Pain with palpation in these areas, and pain that localizes to these areas with physical examination maneuvers, allows the examiner to more predictably narrow the differential diagnosis of the patient's presenting complaint (**Fig. 4**).[10] To aid in narrowing the differential diagnosis, another technique that can be used at this time involves the use of a diagnostic anesthetic injection in differing locations.

A subacromial injection may address subacromial bursitis (associated with LHBT disorders) but would not typically provide relief of pain from primary LHBT disorders, unless there is a rotator cuff tear also present. A glenohumeral injection will provide relief of LHBT anchor pain and intra-articular disorder pain, and it may track to the level of the bicipital groove, depending on inflammation and thickening of the LHBT as it courses distally. Finally, an LHBT sheath injection will provide relief of the LHBT pain, and it may track back to the glenohumeral joint providing relief of intra-articular pain.[10]

The authors agree that when available, ultrasound guidance should be used to verify the location of the injection. The anesthetic of choice, as any of these injections have the potential to reach the glenohumeral joint, should be ropivacaine (Naropin), as it has been shown to be less chondrotoxic than bupivacaine.[13,14]

MUSCULOSKELETAL ULTRASOUND EVALUATION AND INTERVENTION
Overview

Musculoskeletal ultrasound scan can provide immediate visualization of the underlying anatomy of the LHBT and surrounding tissues. Used in trained hands, ultrasound scan can accurately detect fluid swelling within the LHBT sheath, tendinosis of the

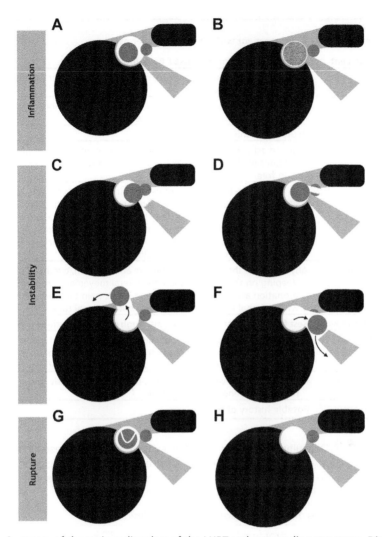

Fig. 3. Summary of the various disorders of the LHBT and surrounding structures. Disorders include (*A*) swelling in the LHBT sheath indicating primary tendinitis, (*B*) thickening and irregularity of the LHBT indicating secondary tendinitis (tendinosis), (*C*) rupture of the subscapularis tendon with LHBT medial subluxation, (*D*) rupture of the medial coracohumeral ligament–superior glenohumeral ligament complex with LHBT medial subluxation, (*E*) rupture of the lateral coracohumeral ligament (and associated supraspinatus anterior fibers) with LHBT lateral dislocation, (*F*) rupture of the medial coracohumeral ligament–superior glenohumeral ligament complex and subscapularis tendon rupture with LHBT medial dislocation, (*G*) partial split tearing of the LHBT, and (*H*) complete rupture with retraction of the LHBT.

LHBT, complete rupture of the LHBT, medial subluxation or dislocation of the LHBT, and associated subscapularis and supraspinatus tendon conditions.[15–23] Ultrasound-guided injection of the LHBT sheath is found to be more accurate than a blind palpation-based approach.[18] However, ultrasound scan does have its limitations. Ultrasound scan is found to be unreliable when detecting partial-thickness tearing

Table 1 Overview of a history that a patient with an LHBT disorder may have	
History Element	**Findings Consistent with LHBT Pathology**
Onset	Insidiously with no inciting event, or after injury, or after repetitive motions of the shoulder
Location	Anterior (in the area of the bicipital groove), with possible radiation to the midsubstance of the biceps muscle
Duration	Acute or chronic
Character	Dull and achy with accentuated episodes of being sharp, complete ruptures may initially present with pain, but may progress to being pain free
Associated symptoms	Pain at rest, mechanical symptoms: popping/snapping/clicking at the anterior shoulder during arc of motion, night time symptoms of pain, cramping of the biceps muscle with strenuous use of the arm, bruising from the middle of the upper arm down toward the elbow, a bulge in the upper arm above the elbow (Popeye deformity) may appear, with an indentation closer to the shoulder
Aggravating factors	Any use of the shoulder, use of the arm at waist level, overhead activities, sleeping on the affected shoulder, lateral movements, supination/pronation activities, resisted elbow flexion, pain that radiates laterally with external rotation and medially with internal rotation
Relieving factors	Rest from aggravating activities, although pain may continue even at rest
X-ray imaging	Normal plan film radiographs of the shoulder, or signs of chronic enthesopathy, superior migration of the humeral head or degenerative changes to the acromioclavicular and glenohumeral joints.
Previous injuries	History of heavy overhead activities, history of previously documented rotator cuff tendinopathy or tear
Social history	Possible history of tobacco use

of the LHBT.[15] Difficulty also arises with the evaluation of an obese or muscular patient, as image resolution decreases with increased depth. Ultrasound scan is also operator dependent and generally requires a great deal of experience with evaluation and guided injection to provide consistent results.

Long Head of Biceps Tendon Ultrasound Protocol/Clinical Case

The author's ultrasound protocol for evaluation of the LHBT involves specific patient positioning and ultrasound probe positioning (**Figs. 5–7**). The different patient and ultrasound positions allow for evaluation of normal anatomy and diagnosis of varying pathologies of the LHBT.

Here is presented a case of a 42-year-old patient who was evaluated for a multiple-year history of anterior shoulder pain with point tenderness in the bicipital groove and a popping sensation noted when lifting objects, which began after a motor vehicle accident 8 years prior. Ultrasound images show swelling in the LHBT sheath and medial subluxation of the LHBT (**Fig. 8**). The patient declined corticosteroid injection and underwent a successful treatment protocol as detailed later in this article.

Ultrasound-Guided Injection/Clinical Case

As previously mentioned, ultrasound-guided injection of the LHBT sheath has been found to be more accurate than a blind palpation-based approach.[18] We present a case of a 54-year-old patient who presented with anterior shoulder pain, accentuated with resisted elbow flexion and active extension of the humerus with the elbow fully

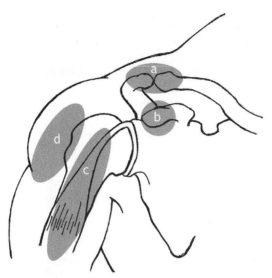

Fig. 4. Shoulder pain locations. (a) Superior pain at the acromioclavicular joint. (b) Anterior pain at the coracoid process. (c) Anterior pain at the bicipital groove radiating to the biceps muscle midbelly. (d) Lateral pain at the greater tuberosity radiating to the deltoid muscle insertion.

extended. He was found to have anterior fascial restriction secondary to scarring over the anterior aspect of the rotator cuff interval, which was causing a tethering effect through the arc of motion. He underwent a steroid injection of the LHBT sheath and hydrodissection procedure of the rotator cuff interval and surrounding tissues, leaving the office pain free **(Fig. 9)**.

Additional Advanced Imaging

There are no clear guidelines for the timing of advanced imaging (MRI, magnetic resonance arthrogram [MRA]) for further delineation of LHBT disorders. However, the authors agree, from a utilization standpoint, that early use of MRI/MRA should be reserved for patients who are young, highly motived exercisers, or elite-level athletes that present with signs of instability and partial or complete rupture. Otherwise, given the potential benefits and success of nonoperative management for most LHBT tendinopathies, a management strategy involving pharmacologic treatment options, ultrasound-guided injections, and multiphase physical rehabilitation should first be used before advanced imaging is considered.

NONOPERATIVE ALGORITHM
Overview

Although there are several articles proposing different nonoperative treatment protocols, there are currently no published studies evaluating the response to nonoperative treatment for LHBT disorders. The authors' approach to comprehensive management of LHBT tendinopathies is algorithm based, built on current evidence from the literature and their own clinical practice **(Fig. 10)**. The algorithm begins with identification of the specific pathologic condition (primary tendonitis, secondary tendonitis [tendinosis], instability, and rupture), moves to pharmacologic modalities and ultrasound-guided injections, reviews a multimodal physical rehabilitation program, and ends

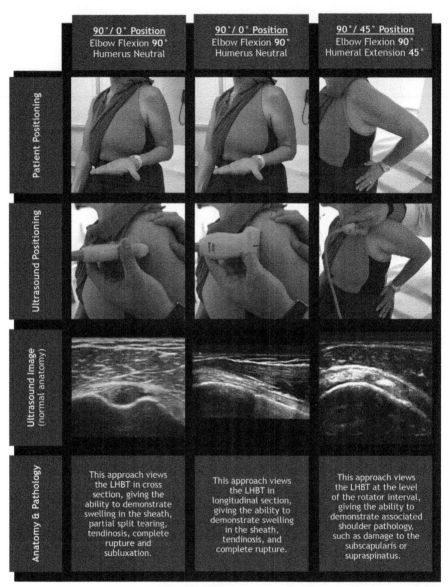

Fig. 5. Ultrasound protocol for LHBT disorders.

with providing guidance after determining the response to the previous interventions. Future studies that evaluate the response to this specific algorithm will provide great insight in determining specific patient populations and LHBT conditions that would benefit from such a protocol.

Note: The superior labrum from anterior to posterior (SLAP) lesion obviously has important implications on LHBT pathology. However, specific management strategies for these SLAP lesions deserve their own review and discussion and are not reviewed in this article to provide for review of treatment protocols for other issues related specifically to the LHBT.

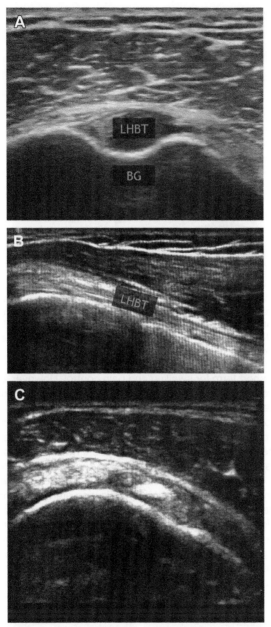

Fig. 6. Anatomic landmarks of images from **Fig. 5.** (*A*) LHBT in short axis. (*B*) LHBT in long axis. (*C*) LHBT at the level of the rotator interval. BG, Bicipital groove.

Nonsteroidal Anti-inflammatory Drugs, Corticosteroid Injections, and Other Modalities

After identification of the underlying pathologic condition of the LHBT, treatment generally begins with activity modification and consideration of nonsteroidal anti-inflammatory drug (NSAID) treatment and/or corticosteroid injection.[3,7,24] NSAIDs

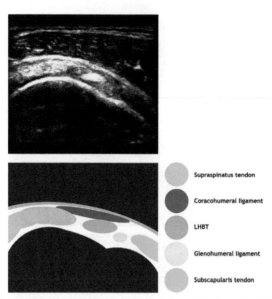

Supraspinatus tendon

Coracohumeral ligament

LHBT

Glenohumeral ligament

Subscapularis tendon

Fig. 7. Ultrasound and pictographic view of the rotator cuff interval. Although it is difficult to view all structures in one view with the same sonographic density because of the concept of anisotropy, careful manipulation of the ultrasound probe can allow visualization of the supraspinatus tendon, the coracohumeral ligament, the LHBT, glenohumeral ligament, and the subscapularis tendon.

can benefit in the short term for swelling and pain control. However, despite the common practice prescribing NSAIDs, there is little evidence that they are efficacious in treating chronic tendon injuries.[24]

A reasonable prescription of an NSAID for initial management of LHBT disorder should include a discussion of the gastrointestinal, renal, and cardiovascular risks of NSAIDS and a prescription for a multiphase physical rehabilitation program.

Use of corticosteroid injections should follow a similar treatment protocol as with NSAIDs. Multiple case reports discuss the risk of tendon rupture with steroid injections, and caution should be exercised when injecting steroid around the LHBT.[24,25] Corticosteroid injections alone will likely provide short-term anti-inflammatory effects for most LHBT disorders. However, they should always be used for short-term pain relief and as an adjunct for the patient to initiate and tolerate a multiphase physical rehabilitation program. Because these injections have the potential to reach the glenohumeral joint, the anesthetic of choice, used in combination with corticosteroid, should be ropivacaine (Naropin), as it is found to be less chondrotoxic than bupivacaine.[13]

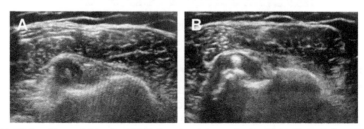

Fig. 8. (A, B) Swelling within the LHBT sheath with medical subluxation of the LHBT.

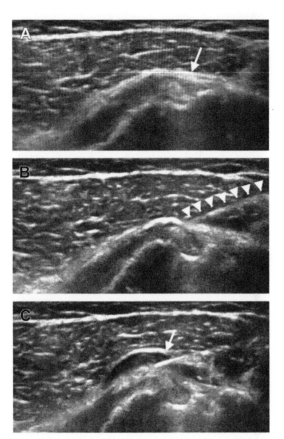

Fig. 9. Ultrasound imaging shows (*A*) thickening of the coracohumeral ligament and capsule, denoted by the arrow. (*B*) The needle, denoted by the arrowheads, can be visualized first injecting into the biceps tendon sheath and then (*C*) being retracted and redirected to address the fascial thickening and restriction. The fascial plane anterior to the coracohumeral ligament and rotator interval capsule can be seen being hydrodissected, denoted by the arrow. The patient left the office pain free with no restriction of motion.

Other modalities that can be used to address LHBT disorders include topical nitroglycerin, iontophoresis, phonophoresis, therapeutic ultrasound scan, extracorporeal shock wave therapy, and low-level laser therapy.[24]

These modalities have been evaluated, but existing medical literature, consisting mostly of small or poorly controlled studies, has demonstrated mixed results.[24,25] Although current medical literature does not support these modalities as first-line treatment, they may be a favorable option for patients as a less invasive and less costly alternative to surgery. The authors recommend using these modalities during phase 1 of the multiphase physical rehabilitation protocol, as discussed later in this article.

Regenerative Injection Therapy for Long Head of Biceps Tendon Disorders

As discussed earlier, ultrasound-guided injections serve an important role in the nonsurgical management of LHBT disorders, and **Fig. 10** lists ultrasound-guided injections as an early intervention strategy. A specific ultrasound-guided therapy

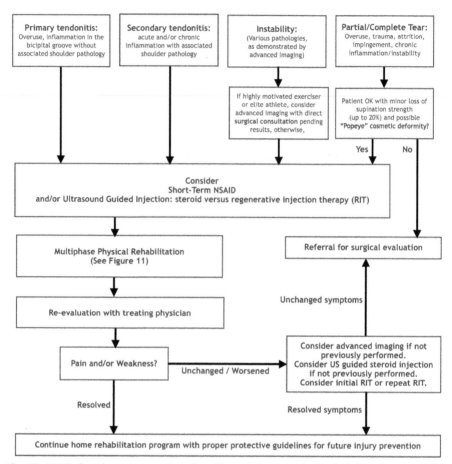

Fig. 10. LHBT disorder nonoperative algorithm. First assess the underlying disorder. Next, determine the need for surgical evaluation versus the appropriate use of NSAIDs or ultrasound-guided injection. Next, progress the patient through a multiphase physical rehabilitation program. The patient will then follow up in the office to determine response to treatment. At that time, continuation of home exercise program versus consideration of additional interventions will be discussed, based on change in symptoms. If a patient progresses through all steps of the algorithm and notes no improvement of pain or weakness with multiple conservative interventions, he or she should progress to surgical evaluation.

protocol, regenerative injection therapy (RIT), uses different injectates to induce an inflammatory response in an attempt to heal and regenerate damaged tissue.[24–28] The choice to perform a RIT varies from patient to patient and condition to condition, and current literature is beginning to thoroughly evaluate these interventions and to standardize treatment protocols for RIT.[20,26–29]

RIT treatments include prolotherapy (dextrose solution, sodium morrhuate), platelet-rich plasma (differing concentrations of platelets, white blood cells, red blood cells, and activated and inactivated platelets), and stem cells (circulating stem cells, adipose derived, bone marrow aspirate, bone marrow aspirate concentrate, amniotic membrane derived).[25,26,28,30]

Indications for RIT include pain impairing athletic performance, connective tissue laxity impairing athletic performance, and pain impairing rest and quality of life.[27]

It is the authors' opinion that, although RIT may induce tissue healing and stimulate regrowth of tissue, RIT alone does not fully address the altered biomechanics or enhance performance. The authors recommend that a multiphase physical rehabilitation program should be performed by every patient who would be a candidate for RIT before the RIT and continued after the RIT. Future research is needed to determine which LHBT disorders respond best to individual or combined RIT and what patient populations are the most suitable candidates for such procedures. The authors recommend that RIT always be performed under ultrasound guidance to document accurate delivery of the injectate.

Multiphase physical rehabilitation

The concept of a multiphase physical rehabilitation program allows for progressive increase in muscle strength while providing protection against further LHBT and associated structure injury during rehabilitation.[1,3,4,6,7,25] However, there is no existing medical literature evaluating any nonoperative physical rehabilitation program for the various LHBT disorders.[25] It is the authors' opinion that nearly every patient with primary or secondary tendonitis, and most patients with instability and partial LHBT tearing, undergo a multiphase physical rehabilitation program before surgical evaluation (or RIT consultation), as many of the symptoms associated with these disorders are likely to be improved through this program (**Fig. 11**).

Treatment follow-up

After progressing a patient through the multiphase physical rehabilitation, it is important to reevaluate the patient for progression of pain, weakness, and mechanical symptoms. At that time, if symptoms are improved, the patient should continue with their home exercise program, and there should be a discussion regarding proper protective guidelines for future injury prevention. If the patient's symptoms are not improved, the authors recommend the following options as next best step on a case-by-case basis:

- Consider advanced imaging if not previously performed.
- Consider ultrasound-guided steroid injection if not previously performed.
- Consider initial RIT or repeat RIT.
- Consider surgical evaluation.

Referral for surgical evaluation

The criteria for surgical evaluation for LHBT and associated disorders includes[25,31]:

- Young, highly motivated exercisers with instability or complete LHBT rupture
- Manual laborers with significant instability or complete LHBT rupture
- Elite-level athletes with instability of complete LHBT rupture
- Any individual with a complete LHBT rupture and is not agreeable with a potential loss of elbow flexion strength (up to 20%) and longstanding "Popeye" deformity
- Any individual who has progressed through all stages of the authors' suggested nonoperative treatment algorithm (see **Fig. 10**) and continues to have symptoms of pain and/or weakness that affects their quality of life

For these patients who have been treated according to the outlined nonoperative treatment algorithm and who meet the above criteria, the authors recommend MRI/MRA

```
┌─────────────────────────────────────────────────────────┐
│                  Rehabilitation Phase 1                  │
│   Goal: Pain management, pain free passive range of      │
│              motion                                      │
│        Avoid: abduction and overhead exercises           │
│                                                          │
│   Wall Walk, Towel Stretches, Pulley Stretches,          │
│   Sleeper Stretch                                        │
│   Additional Modalities: topical nitroglycerin,          │
│   iontophoresis, therapeutic ultrasound ,extracorporeal  │
│   shock wave therapy, low-level laser therapy            │
└─────────────────────────────────────────────────────────┘
```

```
┌─────────────────────────────────────────────────────────┐
│                 Rehabilitation Phase 2:                  │
│             Continue with Phase 1 modalities             │
│                                                          │
│   Goal: Pain free active range of motion, basic          │
│              strengthening                               │
│           Avoid: Overhead resistance                     │
│                                                          │
│   Prone I, T, W, Y arm positioning/ Ceiling punch        │
│   (supine)                                               │
│   Scapular stabilization (not above 90°)                 │
│   Rotator cuff strengthening (IR/ER at 60°)              │
└─────────────────────────────────────────────────────────┘
```

```
┌─────────────────────────────────────────────────────────┐
│                 Rehabilitation Phase 3:                  │
│       Continue with Phase 1 modalities & Phase 2         │
│                    strengthening                         │
│                                                          │
│   Goal: Advance rotator cuff and periscapular strength   │
│   Avoid: Overhead weightlifting, upright rows, wide      │
│   grip bench press                                       │
│                                                          │
│   Bear Hug, Reverse Fly, Rotator cuff strengthening      │
│   (IR/ER at 90°)                                         │
│   Push-Up Progression, Reverse Push-Up Progression       │
│   2 arm plyometric exercises                             │
│                                                          │
│   Weight Training: Hands kept within eyesight, elbows    │
│   bent                                                   │
└─────────────────────────────────────────────────────────┘
```

```
┌─────────────────────────────────────────────────────────┐
│                 Rehabilitation Phase 4:                  │
│       Continue with Phase 1 modalities & Phase 3         │
│                    strengthening                         │
│                                                          │
│   Goal: Return to Activity / Return to Sport             │
│          Work / Sport specific progression               │
└─────────────────────────────────────────────────────────┘
```

Fig. 11. Multiphase physical rehabilitation program. Rehabilitation phase 1 focuses on pain management and pain-free passive range of motion with the inclusion of additional modalities as needed. Rehabilitation phase 2 focuses on pain-free active range of motion with basic strengthening against gravity. Rehabilitation phase 3 focuses on advanced rotator cuff and periscapular strengthening. Rehabilitation phase 4 focuses on return to activity and return to sport. There are also recommendations for activities to avoid during these phases. These are general guidelines and no specific time requirement is placed on these phases.

evaluation (with a 3-T MRI) before surgical consultation to provide the surgeon with the most recent pathology review and to expedite consultation for the patient.

SUMMARY

Diagnosis and nonoperative management of LHBT disorders are categorized as inflammation, instability, and rupture. Specific protocols that address these categories are necessary for comprehensive treatment. Musculoskeletal ultrasound scan can provide real-time imaging of LHBT and associated structure disorders and can provide guidance for increased accuracy of injection. A multiphase physical rehabilitation program allows for progressive increase in muscle strength while possibly providing protection against further LHBT and associated structure injury. RIT may provide significant benefit in the healing and rehabilitation process of LHBT and associated structure disorders; however, further research is needed to define protocols and patient populations likely to benefit from this therapy.

REFERENCES

1. Barber AF, Field LD, Ryu RK. Biceps tendon and superior labrum injuries: decision making. J Bone Joint Surg Am 2007;89(8):1844–55. Available at: http://jbjs.org/content/89/8/1844.
2. Beall DP, Williamson EE, Ly JQ, et al. Association of biceps tendon tears with rotator cuff abnormalities: degree of correlation with tears of the anterior and superior portions of the rotator cuff. Am J Roentgenol 2003;180(3):633–9. Available at: http://www.ajronline.org/doi/abs/10.2214/ajr.180.3.1800633.
3. Allen L. Long head of biceps tendon: anatomy, biomechanics, pathology, diagnosis and management. UNM Orthopaedics Res J 2013;2:21–3. Available at: http://orthopaedics.unm.edu/common/forms/journal-vol2.pdf.
4. Eakin CL, Faber KJ, Hawkins RJ, et al. Biceps tendon disorders in athletes. J Am Acad Orthop Surg 1999;7(5):300–10. Available at: http://www.jaaos.org/content/7/5/300.long.
5. Walch G, Edwards TB, Boulahia A, et al. Arthroscopic tenotomy of the long head of the biceps in the treatment of rotator cuff tears: clinical and radiographic results of 307 cases. J Shoulder Elbow Surg 2005;14(3):238–46. Available at: http://www.jshoulderelbow.org/article/S1058-2746(04)00240-X/abstract.
6. Ryu JH, Pedowitz RA. Rehabilitation of biceps tendon disorders in athletes. Clin Sports Med 2010;29(2):229–46. Available at:http://www.sportsmed.theclinics.com/article/S0278-5919(09)00096-9/abstract.
7. Nho SJ, Strauss EJ, Lenart BA, et al. Long head of the biceps tendinopathy: diagnosis and management. J Am Acad Orthop Surg 2010;18(11):645–56. Available at: http://www.jaaos.org/content/18/11/645.short.
8. Petchprapa CN, Beltran LS, Jazrawi LM, et al. The rotator interval: a review of anatomy, function, and normal and abnormal MRI appearance. AJR Am J Roentgenol 2010;195(3):567–76. Available at: http://www.ajronline.org/doi/abs/10.2214/AJR.10.4406.
9. Bennett WF. Correlation of the SLAP lesion with lesions of the medial sheath of the biceps tendon and intra-articular subscapularis tendon. Indian J Orthop 2009;43(4):342. Available at: http://www.ncbi.nlm.nih.gov/pmc/articles/PMC2762561/.
10. Krupp RJ, Kevern MA, Gaines MD, et al. Long head of the biceps tendon pain: differential diagnosis and treatment. J Orthop Sports Phys Ther 2009;39(2):55–70. Available at: http://www.jospt.org/doi/abs/10.2519/jospt.2009.2802#.VWPqflVViko.
11. Brinks A, Koes BW, Volkers AC, et al. Adverse effects of extra-articular corticosteroid injections: a systematic review. BMC Musculoskelet Disord 2010;11(1):206. Available at: http://link.springer.com/article/10.1186%2F1471-2474-11-206?LI=true.
12. Gill HS, El Rassi G, Bahk MS, et al. Physical examination for partial tears of the biceps tendon. Am J Sports Med 2007;35(8):1334–40. Available at: http://ajs.sagepub.com/content/35/8/1334.short.
13. Piper SL, Kim HT. Comparison of ropivacaine and bupivacaine toxicity in human articular chondrocytes. J Bone Joint Surg Am 2008;90(5):986–91. Available at: http://jbjs.org/content/90/5/986.abstract.

14. Khazzam M, George MS, Churchill RS, et al. Disorders of the long head of biceps tendon. J Shoulder Elbow Surg 2012;21(1):136–45. Available at: http://www.jshoulderelbow.org/article/S1058-2746(11)00312-0/abstract.

15. Armstrong A, Teefey SA, Wu T, et al. The efficacy of ultrasound in the diagnosis of long head of the biceps tendon pathology. J Shoulder Elbow Surg 2006;15(1):7–11. Available at: http://www.sciencedirect.com/science/article/pii/S1058274605001540.

16. Fodor D. Ultrasonography of the normal and pathologic long head of biceps tendon. Available at: http://medultrason.ro/assets/Magazines/Medultrason-2009-vol11-no2/medical-ultrasonography-july-2009-vol-11-no-2-page-45-51.pdf.

17. Moosmayer S, Smith HJ. Diagnostic ultrasound of the shoulder-a method for experts only? Results from an orthopedic surgeon with relative inexperience compared to operative findings. Acta Orthop 2005;76(4):503–8. Available at: http://informahealthcare.com/doi/abs/10.1080/17453670510041484.

18. Hashiuchi T, Sakurai G, Morimoto M, et al. Accuracy of the biceps tendon sheath injection: ultrasound-guided or unguided injection? A randomized controlled trial. J Shoulder Elbow Surg 2011;20(7):1069–73. Available at: http://www.sciencedirect.com/science/article/pii/S1058274611001613.

19. Ptasznik R, Hennessy O. Abnormalities of the biceps tendon of the shoulder: sonographic findings. AJR Am J Roentgenol 1995;164(2):409–14. Available at: http://www.ajronline.org/doi/abs/10.2214/ajr.164.2.7839979.

20. Fullerton BD, Reeves DK. Ultrasonography in regenerative injection (prolotherapy) using dextrose, platelet-rich plasma, and other injectants. Phys Med Rehabil Clin N Am 2010;21(3):585–605. Available at: http://www.pmr.theclinics.com/article/S1047-9651(10)00026-4/pdf.

21. Finnoff JT, Smith J, Peck ER. Ultrasonography of the shoulder. Phys Med Rehabil Clin N Am 2010;21(3):481–507. Available at: http://www.pmr.theclinics.com/article/S1047-9651(10)00016-1/abstract.

22. Lento PH, Strakowski JA. The use of ultrasound in guiding musculoskeletal interventional procedures. Phys Med Rehabil Clin N Am 2010;21(3):559–83. Available at: http://www.sciencedirect.com/science/article/pii/S1047965110000197.

23. Nichols AW. Complications associated with the use of corticosteroids in the treatment of athletic injuries. Clin J Sport Med 2005;15(5):E370. Available at: http://journals.lww.com/cjsportsmed/Abstract/2005/09000/Complications_Associated_With_the_Use_of.16.aspx.

24. Childress MA, Beutler A. Management of chronic tendon injuries. Am Fam Physician 2013;87(7):486. Available at: http://www.ncbi.nlm.nih.gov/pubmed/23547590.

25. Andres BM, Murrell GA. Treatment of tendinopathy: what works, what does not, and what is on the horizon. Clin Orthop Relat Res 2008;466(7):1539–54. Available at: http://link.springer.com/article/10.1007/s11999-008-0260-1#page-1.

26. Mautner K, Blazuk J. Where do injectable stem cell treatments apply in treatment of muscle, tendon, and ligament injuries? PM R 2015;7(4):S33–40. Available at: http://www.sciencedirect.com/science/article/pii/S1934148215000106.

27. Reeves DK, Fullerton BD, Topol G. Evidence-based regenerative injection therapy (prolotherapy) in sports medicine. The sports medicine resource manual. Amsterdam, Netherlands: Saunders (Elsevier); 2008. p. 611–9. Available at: http://www.houstonsportsdoctor.com/pdf/sports-medicine-resource-manual2008.pdf.

28. Moon YL, Ha SH, Lee YK, et al. Comparative studies of Platelet-Rich Plasma (PRP) and prolotherapy for proximal biceps tendinitis. Clin Shoulder Elbow 2011;14(2):153–8. Available at: http://www.koreamed.org/SearchBasic.php?RID=1133CISE/2011.14.2.153&DT=1.

29. Finnoff JT, Fowler SP, Lai JK, et al. Treatment of chronic tendinopathy with ultrasound-guided needle tenotomy and platelet-rich plasma injection. PM R 2011;3(10):900–11. Available at: http://www.sciencedirect.com/science/article/pii/S1934148211003637.

30. Mautner K, Malanga GA, Smith J, et al. A call for a standard classification system for future biologic research: The rationale for new PRP nomenclature. PM R 2015;7(4):S53–9. Available at: http://www.sciencedirect.com/science/article/pii/S1934148215000763.

31. Pugach S, Pugach IZ. When is a conservative approach best for proximal biceps tendon rupture? J Fam Pract 2013;62(3):134–6. Available at: http://skin.gcnpublishing.com/fileadmin/jfp_archive/pdf/6203/6203JFP_Article3.pdf.

The Painful Long Head of the Biceps Brachii

Nonoperative Treatment Approaches

Kevin E. Wilk, PT, DPT[a,b,c,]*,
Todd R. Hooks, PT, ATC, OCS, SCS, NREMT-1, CSCS, CMTPT[d,e]

KEYWORDS

- Rehabilitation • Shoulder • Elbow • Biceps

KEY POINTS

- Abnormality involving the long head of the biceps has a variety of clinical conditions affecting either the tendon or the supporting tissues.
- The long head of the biceps tendon can be a primary source of pain or a secondary source of pain as a result of shoulder dysfunction.
- A comprehensive evaluation to determine the causative factors is critical in developing an appropriate treatment program.
- Incorporating applied stresses and forces in a systematic application via functional and sport-specific training ensures a proper return to prior level of function.

Pain associated with the long head of the biceps (LHB) brachii seems to be increasingly recognized in the past 4 to 5 years. The LHB has long been considered a troublesome pain generator in the shoulder. Abnormality involving the LHB brachii has long been an area of debate, with Codman[1] in 1934 even questioning the specificity of the diagnosis of biceps tendinitis. Biceps tendon abnormality is often associated with rotator cuff impingement.[2] Shoulder pain originating from the biceps tendon can be debilitating, causing a severe decrease in shoulder function.[3–7] As a result of the frequent clinical presentation of biceps pain, there is currently a great deal of interest regarding the diagnosis, treatment, and prevention of biceps abnormality. This article describes a classification system of LHB pain and discusses nonoperative treatment concepts and techniques for the painful LHB.

[a] Champion Sports Medicine, A Physiotherapy Associates Clinic, 805 Street Vincent's Drive G100, Birmingham, AL 35205, USA; [b] Tampa Bay Rays Baseball Team, 400 N Tampa Street, Tampa, FL 33602, USA; [c] Physical Therapy Programs, Marquette University, Milwaukee, WI 53201-1881, USA; [d] New Orleans Pelicans Basketball Team, 5800 Airline Drive Metairie, New Orleans, LA 70003, USA; [e] Myopain Seminars, 4405 East-West Highway, Suite 404, Bethesda, MD 20814, USA
* Corresponding author. 805 St Vincent's Drive, G-100, Birmingham, AL 35205.
E-mail address: kwilkpt@hotmail.com

Clin Sports Med 35 (2016) 75–92
http://dx.doi.org/10.1016/j.csm.2015.08.012
0278-5919/16/$ – see front matter © 2016 Elsevier Inc. All rights reserved.

FUNCTION

There exists much controversy regarding the function of the proximal segment of the LHB brachii. The biceps brachii functions at both the shoulder and the elbow, and although there is general agreement that it is a strong supinator of the forearm and weak flexor of the elbow, there is, however, much controversy regarding its function in the shoulder due to contradictory experimental findings. The LHB is thought to function as a humeral head depressor and is also thought to provide stabilization of the glenohumeral joint. Simulated contractions of the LHB performed in cadaveric shoulders have shown significantly decreased anterior, superior, and inferior translation of the humeral head.[8] Biomechanical analysis has demonstrated that the LHB functions to provide anterior stabilization with the glenohumeral joint in abduction and external rotation (ER) with increased contribution noted with anterior instability.[9] Rodosky and colleagues[10] showed via simulated contractions of the biceps in the cadaveric shoulder that the LHB provides resistance to torsional forces with the shoulder in the abducted and externally rotated position, thus providing anterior stability of the glenohumeral joint. The investigators also noted increased strain and less torsional rigidity with detachment of the biceps-labral complex.

Electromyographic (EMG) studies of the LHB remain controversial. Sakurai and colleagues[11] demonstrated activity of the LHB in stabilizing the humeral head, while Levy and colleagues[12] noted that the LHB served as a functional stabilizer only during elbow and forearm activity. Biomechanical analysis during pitching has revealed that the biceps is predominantly active in elbow flexion during arm cocking and during follow-through to decelerate the forearm in order to prevent hyperextension of the elbow.[13] Similarly, Rojas and colleagues[14] noted greater biceps activity during windmill pitching as compared with overhead throwing.

Classification of Long Head of the Biceps Pain and Pathophysiology

The authors have classified LHB pain into 6 specific categories (**Box 1**) based on the pathophysiology and clinical presentation: traumatic injuries, instability, tendinopathy, biomechanical (scapular dysfunction, glenohumeral joint hypermobility), capsular involvement, and superior labral anterior posterior (SLAP) lesions. Although all of these conditions may present with shoulder pain, the pathogenesis, patient population, and treatment will vary.

Traumatic injuries

Long head of the biceps tendon (LHBT) ruptures commonly occur as a result of the degenerative process as a result of tendon instability or impingement. Ruptures

---

Box 1
Classification of long head biceps brachii pain

Traumatic injuries

Instability

Tendinopathies
  Tendonitis
  Tendinosis

Biomechanical dysfunction
  Scapular dysfunction
  Glenohumeral joint hypermobility

Capsular involvement

SLAP lesions

involving the LHBT are more frequent than those of the short head or the distal tendon, representing 96% of all ruptures.[15] The ruptures usually occur at the tendon's origin or as it exits the bicipital groove near the musculotendinous junction.[16] Rupture of the LHBT normally creates a Popeye deformity as the muscle belly moves distally; however, a vincula, adhesion, or hypertrophy of the tendon can prevent this distal migration.[17] These injuries are most common in individuals older than 50 years of age, and they are often associated with biceps tendinitis, which can lead to degeneration of the biceps tendon, causing rupture with minimal trauma.[15,16,18]

Instability

The biceps is secured as it travels from the intra-articular space into the bicipital groove by the biceps reflection pulley, which is formed by the coracohumeral ligament, superior glenohumeral ligament (SGHL), and fibers from both the subscapularis and the supraspinatus tendons.[19] Four different types of lesions have been observed arthroscopically: isolated SGHL (type I), SGHL lesion and partial articular-sided supraspinatus tendon tear (type II), SGHL lesion and deep surface tear of the subscapularis tendon (type III), and a lesion of the SGHL combined with a partial articular-sided supraspinatus and subscapularis tendon tear (type IV).[19] Braun and colleagues[20] conducted a prospective study of 229 patients undergoing shoulder arthroscopy and noted a significant correlation between pulley lesions and SLAP tears, LHB, and rotator cuff abnormality. Distribution of the pulley system can be due to either a traumatic episode or a degeneration that is often associated with rotator cuff abnormality.[21,22] Lesions of the pulley can be a result of contact with the posterosuperior labrum in the late cocking phase of throwing[23] as well as stresses that incur within the tendon with the arm at end range of ER and abduction position that can place stress on the pulley system.[19,24]

Subcoracoid impingement, defined as the subcoracoid bursa and subscapularis tendon impinging between the coracoid and lesser tuberosity, has also been described as a potential cause of degeneration of the pulley sling and subscapularis tendon insertion.[22] Narrowing of the coracohumeral interval, the distance between the humeral head and the coracoid tip, has been shown to be related to LHB and rotator cuff abnormality.[22]

Following a lesion of the pulley, the LHB becomes unstable, causing degenerative changes of the tendon and the surrounding tissues. Instability of the tendon most frequently occurs medially, which typically affects the subscapularis tendon. Two variations of instability can occur: subluxation and dislocation. Subluxation is the most common, with these patients having more subjective complaints of pain. Patients with dislocations often have pseudoparalysis as a result of the associated rotator cuff abnormality.[25]

Biceps Tendinopathy

Biceps tendonitis is inflammation of the LHBT and is most often a result of other pathologic conditions at the shoulder, including rotator cuff lesions and impingement syndrome, and is therefore often considered a secondary condition.[26] Bicipital tendonitis presenting as a primary condition is rare and has been estimated to occur in only 5% of all cases.[27] Rotator cuff abnormality has been associated with LHBT tendonitis, as Chen and colleagues[28] reported 76% of rotator cuff tears had associated LHBT tendonitis, while Gill and colleagues[29] found 85% of patients with partial rotator cuff tears had associated LHBT tendinopathy. Chronic tenosynovitis can cause enlargement of the tendon and thickening of the tendon sheath, which has been described as the hourglass biceps.[30] As a result, the tendon can become entrapped within the groove as the intra-articular portion of the tendon gets incarcerated within the joint, creating mechanical symptoms of pain and locking. Tendons have a 7.5 times lower oxygen uptake than skeletal muscles, potentially decreasing the healing capacity.[31] As a result, tendinosis can occur due to chronic degeneration without the presence of inflammation.

Biomechanical Dysfunction

Proper positioning of the scapula is important in normal upper extremity function. Scapular dyskinesis is abnormal positioning or motion of the scapula during coupled scapulohumeral movements.[32] Scapular dyskinesis has also been associated with subacromial impingement[33] and can affect biceps function and should therefore be assessed in the evaluation of biceps abnormality.[32] The commonly seen presentation of a rounded shoulder and forward head position reduces the subacromial space.[34] Because of an altered length-tension relationship, this position can cause muscle weakness/inhibition of the posterior scapular muscles, particularly the rhomboids and lower trapezius. Decreased flexibility or adaptive shortening of the pectoralis minor can also occur due to scapular malpositioning.

Secondary LHB abnormality can develop from glenohumeral instability, which has been shown to cause increased rotator cuff and biceps activity in order to provide anterior stability of the glenohumeral joint.[35,36] In addition, increased humeral translation and resultant internal impingement can occur as a result of the subtle glenohumeral instability that is often noted in the overhead athlete. This microinstability can cause fraying of the posterior rotator cuff and superior labral biceps anchor. Tendon degeneration or anchor failure can occur as a result of these stresses.

Capsular Involvement

The synovial lining of the biceps tendon sheath is continuous with the glenohumeral joint; therefore, synovitis of the glenohumeral joint capsule can cause pain into the LHB as a result of this relationship. Furthermore, inflammation of the glenohumeral joint capsule can cause pain in the LHB as a result of capsular mechanoreceptor input.

Superior Labral Anterior Posterior Lesions

SLAP lesions can occur as a result of several mechanisms, including a fall on an outstretched hand,[37] tensile forces on the biceps anchor as a result of eccentric biceps contraction during the throwing motion,[38] or a peel-back mechanism as the arm is maximally externally rotated during throwing.[39] Synder and colleagues[37] have classified these injuries into 4 types, with type II and IV SLAP lesions resulting in instability of the biceps anchor. SLAP lesions have been reported to have a strong correlation with glenohumeral instability,[10,39] rotator cuff tears,[40] and scapular dyskinesis.[39]

CLINICAL EXAMINATION

The symptoms associated with biceps abnormality can often be difficult to distinguish from that of other shoulder abnormality and often occur in conjunction with other pathologic conditions of the shoulder. Biceps tendonitis commonly presents with anterior shoulder pain with tenderness noted at the bicipital groove and a positive Speed test. However, when using these criteria, 90% of all painful shoulders could be considered as having biceps tendinitis.[41] As a result, it is important to be cognitive of other potential causative factors when considering the biceps as a source of pain. Therefore, a complete and comprehensive evaluation is needed to determine the causative factors.

History

Patients commonly present with chronic pain in the proximal anterior shoulder that may extend into the belly of the biceps muscle. The patient is usually young or middle aged with a history of pain that increases with activity and decreases with rest. Symptoms commonly increase at night as the patient lies either on the affected arm (compressive loading) or in a supine position (decreased venous return and shoulder in an extended position).

Although the term bicipital tendonitis is often used, it is a misnomer because histologic inflammatory changes within the tendon are rarely seen, representing approximately 5% of all cases.[27,42] Patients presenting with peritendinitis will have pain that is worse with activities that are accentuated with overhead sports and movements away from the body. Palpation of the biceps tendon is best performed with the arm in approximately 10° of internal rotation (IR), which positions the biceps tendon anteriorly with pain noted with palpation 3 inches below the acromion.[43,44] Although it will not differentiate biceps tendinopathy from biceps instability, if a biceps lesion is present, this groove tenderness will migrate with rotation of the arm. This palpation with movement strategy can allow the examiner to differentiate bicipital abnormality from other conditions such as subdeltoid bursitis or impingement, because symptoms in the latter are often more diffuse and will not migrate with arm movement. Special tests aimed at the direct evaluation of the biceps such as Speed test[45] and Yergason test[46] can be useful. Because of the concomitant presentation of biceps abnormality with SLAP and rotator cuff abnormality, special tests such as the biceps tension sign[37] and the active compression test[47] are warranted to evaluate the status of these structures.

Tendinosis can be difficult to discern from peritendinitis because the patient will have similar subjective complaints, and the clinical examination will be similar. However, tendinosis is a result of tendon degeneration, and thus, the patient will often report pain at rest. The authors also perform passive flexion and extension of the elbow with the aim of allowing the tendon to slide within the tendon sheath; this moves the patient's point tenderness as the tendon translates within the sheath. Rupture of the biceps tendon is frequently associated with tendon degeneration, most often occurring at the tendon's origin or at the myotendinous junction as it exits the bicipital groove,[16,18] which will result in the formation of the Popeye deformity.

Biceps instability can be a result of different types of lesions involving the SGHL, subscapularis, or supraspinatus.[19] Clinical tests to evaluate for the presence of a pulley lesion causing instability of the biceps include the Biceps Instability Test[3] and Ludington test,[48] which is performed by having the patient place his or her hands behind the head and contract the biceps as the examiner palpates in the groove to detect subluxation. Assessing the stability of the glenohumeral joint with such tests as the anterior and posterior drawer[49] or the apprehension test[50] can assess for the presence of hypermobility.

NONOPERATIVE TREATMENT

The nonoperative rehabilitation program is based on the clinical examination of each patient. This program is adaptable to allow the treatment of both traumatic and atraumatic injuries. Treatment of biceps abnormality will often focus on an associated shoulder dysfunction, including rotator cuff tendinopathy, glenohumeral instability, subacromial impingement, and SLAP lesions.[35,51–53]

PHASE 1: ACUTE PHASE

The goals in the first phase of treatment are to diminish pain and inflammation, normalize motion and muscle balance, restore baseline dynamic stability, and correct postural adaptations. The patient may be prescribed nonsteroidal anti-inflammatory medication and/or a local corticosteroid injection, which have been shown to provide pain relief with biceps tendinopathy.[41] In the presence of more significant biceps tendinopathy, the patient may not respond to this injection and may require an injection directly into the tendon sheath.[41,54,55] Barber and colleagues[53] described injections directly into the glenohumeral joint to avoid any potential complications of direct tendon injection, to administer the medication directly to the often-irritated intra-articular portion of the biceps. In the acute phases of treatment of peritendinitis, the rehabilitation specialist will use local modalities to diminish pain and inflammation, such as ice, laser (**Fig. 1**), and iontophoresis (**Fig. 2**). The clinician can decrease pain and muscle guarding by stimulating type 1 and 2 mechanoreceptors with active assistive range of motion (AAROM), light stretching activities, and grade 1 and 2 joint mobilizations.[56–58] A 23% reduction in EMG with a 32% resultant decrease in ER force production has been reported in a painful shoulder.[59] Consequently, because of the interwoven relationship of the rotator cuff and the biceps, pain relief is sought during this phase of treatment. However, in the presence of a tendinosis, the treatment will focus on increasing local circulation to augment tendon healing. Therefore, the clinician may use moist heat, laser, and ultrasound to increase local circulation/soft tissue extensibility and promote healing.

Mechanical stimulation using dry needling can be included to augment the healing in the treatment of biceps tendinopathy.[60–64] Trigger points have been shown to cause a decrease in local blood flow[65,66] and create a subsequent hypoxic environment that can contribute to tendon dysrepair.[67] In addition, trigger points have been shown to be a source of nociceptive input[68,69] and contribute to abnormal muscle activation patterns.[70] Dry needling has been demonstrated to increase blood flow via local vasodilation[61–63,71] and collagen proliferation by increasing fibroblastic activity.[60,64] Repeated fenestration of the tendon by needling mechanically causes bleeding by disrupting the local scar tissue.[72,73] The bleeding stimulates growth factors by mediating transforming growth factor-β and basic fibroblastic growth factor.[63,74] These growth factors stimulate healing by increasing matrix synthesis and promoting cellular proliferation[75] to aid in the remodeling of the tendon and restoring its mechanical properties.[76] Dry needling has also been shown to have central effects via activation of the

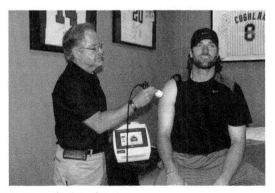

Fig. 1. Therapeutic laser applied to the LHB.

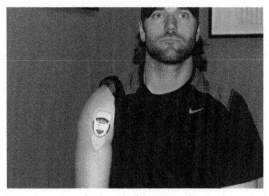

Fig. 2. Iontophoresis treatment applied to the biceps tendon to decrease local inflammation.

descending pain inhibitory systems, cortex, hypothalamus, and the inactivation of the limbic system,[77–81] rendering this treatment useful in the reduction of pain. Therefore, a thorough assessment for the presence of trigger points in the biceps and the surrounding musculature is warranted to aid in the treatment of bicipital pathologic conditions (**Fig. 3**).

The clinician should restore normal range of motion (ROM) for the shoulder and elbow joint by incorporating AAROM, passive range of motion, manual stretches, and joint mobilization techniques. Ensuring full physiologic mobility of the biceps via stretching exercises should be included to decrease tension in the tendon and the musculotendinous junction. The overhead athlete will typically exhibit a loss of IR. A loss of IR of 18° in the throwing shoulder has been associated with shoulder and elbow injuries.[82,83] Wright and colleagues[84] have also reported an average loss of 7° elbow extension in professional baseball pitchers.

Proper mobility and stability of the scapula are essential for normal function of the upper extremity. Scapular positioning has been shown to contribute to subacromial impingement,[33] with a decreased subacromial space noted as the scapula moves into a protracted position.[34] Because of an altered length-tension relationship, this position can cause muscle weakness of the posterior scapular muscles, particularly the rhomboids and lower trapezius. In addition, a protracted scapula may result in increased biceps muscle activity and muscle spasm. Decreased flexibility or adaptive shortening of the pectoralis minor can occur due to scapular malpositioning. Stretching exercises aimed at the pectoralis minor muscle can be performed as the patient places the scapula in a retracted and posteriorly tilted position with 30° of shoulder flexion as the humerus is maintained in abduction and ER.[85,86] Corrective positioning

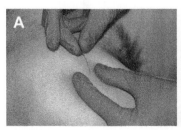
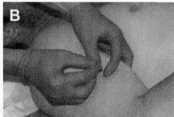

Fig. 3. Dry needling treatment to (*A*) LHB brachii, and (*B*) muscle belly of the biceps brachii trigger point.

of the scapula has been shown to open the subacromial space as well as increase the strength of the supraspinatus in patients with subacromial impingement.[87,88] Tactile stimulation provided by specially designed postural shirts can be worn during activities of daily living and during the rehabilitation program to improve scapular positioning (**Fig. 4**).

In addition, for sympathetic pain relief, the clinician can tape or brace the biceps brachii in an attempt to reduce pain during activities of daily living or rehabilitation exercises. Examples include Kinesio taping and use of a Cho-Pat strap.

Strengthening exercises are incorporated in the first phase of rehabilitation aimed at restoring muscle balance and retarding muscle atrophy.[89,90] Clinical judgment can dictate the initiation of either isometrics in the presence of excessive pain or soreness, which will be progressed to isotonics as tolerated. Rhythmic stabilization (RS) exercises are performed for the biceps and triceps and can also be performed at the shoulder by performing internal and external rotation beginning with the arm at 30° of abduction and with the arm placed at approximately 100° of elevation and 10° of horizontal abduction. This balanced position is beneficial because the deltoid and rotator cuff resultant force vectors provide a centralized compression of the humeral head.[91,92] The authors attempt to improve glenohumeral joint dynamic stabilization through rotator cuff muscle efficiency, thus decreasing the demands of the LHB to stabilize the humeral head in the glenoid fossa.

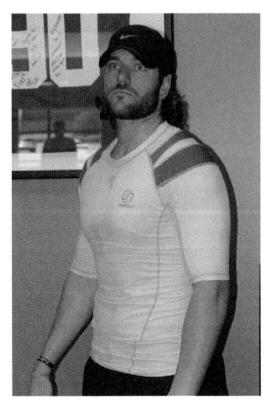

Fig. 4. A postural cueing shirt designed to give tactile stimulation for optimal positioning. (Intelliskin, Huntington Beach, CA.)

Microtrauma or macrotrauma can affect proprioceptive awareness; therefore, drills to increase the neurosensory properties of the joint capsule and surrounding soft tissue should be included in the early phases of rehabilitation.[93,94] RS drills improve proximal stability by performing exercises for the rotator cuff and the scapulothoracic musculature and can be progressed to proprioceptive neuromuscular facilitation (PNF) patterns while incorporating RSs aimed at enhancing proprioception and dynamic stability.[89,90,93–96] Weight-bearing drills, such as weight shifts, wall pushups, and quadrupled exercises, aimed at stimulating the articular mechanoreceptors and restoring proprioception can also be included in the first phase of treatment.[90,97,98] Utilization of a full prone plank can be effective for core stabilization and coactivation of shoulder muscles. Efficient transfer of kinetic energy and effective proximal stability are important for upper extremity overhead activities such as throwing. Core exercises are also included to provide proper stability, mobility, and postural education.

In addition, light biceps brachii strengthening exercises are initiated during this phase. The authors gradually begin with light Theraband biceps curls in the seated position with the elbow supported by the patient's leg. The patient is instructed to emphasize the eccentric phase during the exercise in an attempt to stimulate collagen synthesis and organization.

PHASE 2: INTERMEDIATE PHASE

The intermediate phase is designed to continue to progress the strengthening program; increase flexibility, mobility, and ROM of the elbow and shoulder joint complex; and further enhance the patient's neuromuscular control. Strengthening exercises are progressed in this phase to include more aggressive isotonics aimed at restoring optimal muscle force couples by performing the Thrower's 10 program,[97] which is designed to restore muscle balance and is based on EMG data.[13,99–106]

The clinician will continue to progress the strengthening program to include manual resistance drills and can also include concentric and eccentric contractions and incorporate RS drills during the exercise. Neuromuscular drills are progressed by performing stabilization holds at the end ROMs. In addition, PNF exercises that include RS drills in various degrees of movement are performed throughout the patient's available ROM. These exercises and drills serve to improve dynamic stability and local muscle endurance.

Optimal scapular function is crucial to provide proximal stability and allow for efficient distal arm mobility and optimal shoulder function.[107–110] The scapular retractors, protractors, and depressors are commonly emphasized because of the inherent muscle weakness commonly seen due to poor posture and deconditioning. The authors implement a program designed with specific exercises to isolate weak muscles, improve muscle activation, and normalize the muscular force couples of the scapulothoracic joint and stimulate neuromuscular control.[90] These exercises include wall slides (serratus anterior, **Fig. 5**), lower trapezius modified robbery (**Fig. 6**), prone horizontal abduction (rhomboids/middle trapezius, **Fig. 7**), prone row into ER, side-lying scapular neuromuscular control exercise (**Fig. 8**), and prone full can.

Isolated biceps brachii strengthening is progressed during this phase; during this phase, the amount of resistance is increased and a longer eccentric phase is used to produce more load onto the biceps tendon. In addition, brachioradialis, triceps, and wrist extensors/flexors are all exercised as well.

Closed kinetic chain exercises are progressed to include proprioceptive drills, such as table pushups on a tilt board or ball. These exercises have been shown to generate increased upper and middle trapezius, and serratus anterior activity as compared with

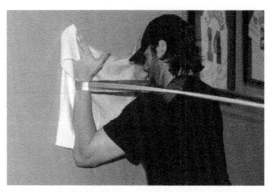

Fig. 5. Wall slide exercise to facilitate serratus anterior activity.

a standard pushup.[111] Stabilization drills can be progressed to include placing the hand on a small ball against a wall performed in a RS drill (**Fig. 9**). Progression from a full prone plank to a side plank can be beneficial and challenging to the core and scapular musculature.

PHASE 3: ADVANCED STRENGTHENING PHASE

The goals of treatment during phase 3 are to initiate aggressive strengthening exercises and functional drills, progress muscular endurance and power, and prepare for a return to sporting activity. Muscle fatigue has been shown to decrease neuromuscular control, diminish proprioception, and alter scapular positioning.[112,113] The Advanced Thrower's 10 program was designed to incorporate alternate movement patterns of the upper extremity to further challenge the patient's neuromuscular control and restore muscle symmetry and balance and improve muscular endurance.[114] The sustained holds that are incorporated into this program are designed to challenge the patient to maintain an isometric position while performing a reciprocal isotonic movement with the opposite upper extremity. These exercises are usually performed in 3 alternating sets with the first set performed with bilateral isotonic movement, then unilateral isotonic movement with contralateral sustained hold, followed by alternating isotonic/sustained hold sequencing. In addition, the patient can perform these

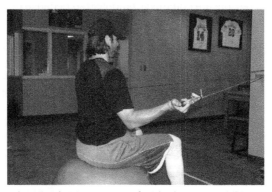

Fig. 6. Activation and strengthening exercise for the lower trapezius muscle, referred to as the modified robbery exercise.

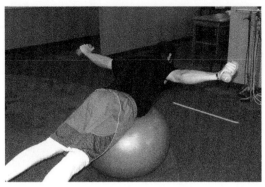

Fig. 7. Prone horizontal abduction performed bilaterally on a Swiss ball to incorporate core stabilization (this exercise is often referred to as prone T's).

exercises on a stability ball to further challenge the core. Manual resistance provided by the clinician can be implemented to augment muscle co-contraction and improve muscular endurance of the shoulder and core.

Neuromuscular control drills are progressed to include side-lying ER with manual resistance. Concentric and eccentric ER is performed as the clinician provides resistance, including RS at end range. These drills can also be progressed to being performed standing using exercise tubing at 0° and finally at 90° abduction.

Eccentric exercises are included in the rehabilitation program particularly in the treatment of biceps tendinosis. In the overhead athlete, the biceps muscle is an important stabilizer during the follow-through phase. Elbow eccentrics can be performed with manual resistance, dumbbells, or elastic tubing to emphasize both slow- and fast-speed contractions. Strengthening exercises are further progressed to include weight machines to further increase strength and power; traditionally, the authors focus on training on the posterior scapula using seated rows and latissimus dorsi pull-downs.

It is important for the patient to continue to perform postural correction exercises during this phase. These exercises would include corner stretches for pectoralis minor tightness, wall circles for posture and lower trapezius activation, and continuation of the scapular muscle strengthening exercises listed above in phase 2.

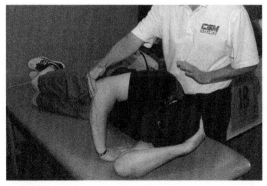

Fig. 8. Side-lying neuromuscular control drills for the scapula using tactile and manual resistance.

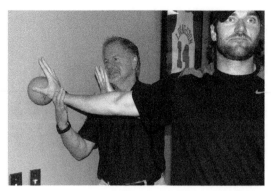

Fig. 9. Dynamic stability training with the hand placed onto a ball to provide compressive forces into the glenohumeral joint while the arm is in the scapular plane as the clinician provides RSs.

An interval sports program can be introduced during the third phase.[115] These programs (golf, tennis, football, baseball, softball, and others) were designed to gradually introduce quantity, intensity, and duration of sporting activities to allow an athlete to return to sporting activities while minimizing the recurrence of injury and pain with activities.

PHASE 4: RETURN TO ACTIVITY PHASE

Phase 4 of the rehabilitation program allows the patient to continue to progress with functional activities and drills that are designed to return the patient to his or her prior level of functional activities. The criterion to initiate this phase of treatment includes full ROM, no pain or tenderness, and a satisfactory clinical examination. Patients are encouraged to maintain and continue to improve upper extremity and core strengthening, flexibility, and neuromuscular drills. Usually athletic patients are placed on the Thrower's 10 program to maintain shoulder strength and flexibility during their competitive season. During this return to activity phase, it is critical for the patient to continue their strengthening, activation, and postural exercises to maintain proper posture and body awareness.

SUMMARY

The LHB has gained recent attention due to its association with shoulder dysfunction and its potential for pain generation. LHB abnormality often occurs concomitantly with other shoulder conditions, and as a result, making a diagnosis can often be difficult. It is imperative that the clinician is able to accurately recognize all underlying causative factors to establish a successful nonoperative rehabilitation program. Based on the abnormality, the rehabilitation program will focus on restoring dynamic stability, restoring muscular endurance, addressing postural adaptations, and providing the appropriate stimulation to augment the healing response to the LHBT.

REFERENCES

1. Codman EA. The shoulder. Boston: Thomas Todd; 1934.
2. Neer CS II. Anterior acromioplasty for the chronic impingement syndrome in the shoulder. J Bone Joint Surg Am 1972;54:41–50.

3. Abbott LC, Saunders LB de CM. Acute traumatic dislocation of the tendon of the long head of biceps brachii: report of 6 cases with operative findings. Surgery 1939;6:817–40.
4. Becker DA, Cofield RH. Tenodesis of the long head of the biceps brachii for chronic bicipital tendinitis. Long-term results. J Bone Joint Surg Am 1989; 71(3):376–81.
5. DePalma AF, Callery GE. Bicipital tenosynovitis. Clin Orthop 1954;3:69–85.
6. Neviaser TJ. The role of the biceps tendon in the impingement syndrome. Orthop Clin North Am 1987;18(3):433–8.
7. Post M, Benca P. Primary tendinitis of the long head of the biceps. Clin Orthop Relat Res 1989;246:117–25.
8. Pagnani MJ, Deng XH, Warren FR, et al. Role of the long head of the biceps brachii in glenohumeral stability: a biomechanical study in cadaver. J Shoulder Elbow Surg 1996;5:255–62.
9. Itoi E, Kuechle DK, Newman SR, et al. Stabilizing function of the biceps in stable and unstable shoulders. J Bone Joint Surg Br 1993;75:546–50.
10. Rodosky MW, Harner CD, Fu FH. The role of the long head of the biceps muscle and superior glenoid labrum in anterior stability of the shoulder. Am J Sports Med 1994;22:121–30.
11. Sakurai G, Tomita Y, Nakagaki K, et al. Role of long head of biceps brachii in rotator cuff tendon failure: an EMG study. J Shoulder Elbow Surg 1996;5:S135.
12. Levy AS, Kelly BT, Lintner SA, et al. Function of the long head of the biceps at the shoulder: electromyographic analysis. J Shoulder Elbow Surg 2001;10:250–5.
13. Jobe FW, Moynes DR, Tibone JE, et al. An EMG analysis of the shoulder in pitching. A second report. Am J Sports Med 1984;12:218–20.
14. Rojas IL, Provencher MT, Bhatia S, et al. Biceps activity during windmill softball pitching: injury implications and comparison with overhand throwing. Am J Sports Med 2009;37:558–65.
15. Carter AN, Erickson SM. Proximal biceps tendon rupture: primarily an injury of middle age. Phys Sportsmed 1999;27:95–101.
16. Rowe CR. The shoulder. New York: Churchill Livingstone; 1988.
17. Johson LL, Bays BM, van Dyk GE. Vincula of the biceps tendon in the glenohumeral joint: an arthroscopic and anatomic study. J Shoulder Elbow Surg 1992;1:162–8.
18. Warren RF. Lesions of the long head of the biceps tendon. Instr Course Lect 1985;34:204–9.
19. Habermeyer P, Magosch P, Pritsch M, et al. Anterosuperior impingement of the shoulder as a result of pulley lesions: a prospective arthroscopic study. J Shoulder Elbow Surg 2004;13:5–12.
20. Braun S, Horan MP, Elser F, et al. Lesions of the biceps pulley. Am J Sports Med 2011;4(4):790–5.
21. Le Huec JC, Schaeverbeke T, Moinard M, et al. Traumatic tear of the rotator interval. J Shoulder Elbow Surg 1996;5:41–6.
22. Gerber C, Sevesta A. Impingement of the deep surface of the subscapularis tendon and the reflection pulley on the anterosuperior glenoid rim: a preliminary report. J Shoulder Elbow Surg 2000;9:483–90.
23. Choi CH, Kim SK, Jang WC, et al. Biceps pulley impingement. Arthroscopy 2004;20(Suppl 2):80–3.
24. Lafosse L, Reiland Y, Baier GP, et al. Anterior and posterior instability of the long head of the biceps tendon in rotator cuff tears: a new classification based on arthroscopic observations. Arthroscopy 2007;23:73–80.

25. Walsh G, Nové-Josserand L, Boileau P, et al. Subluxations and dislocations of the tendon of the long head of the biceps. J Shoulder Elbow Surg 1998;7:100–8.
26. Maier D, Jaeger M, Suedkamp NP, et al. Stabilization of the long head of the biceps tendon in the context of early repair of traumatic subscapularis tendon tears. J Bone Joint Surg Am 2007;89:1763–9.
27. Favorito PJ, Harding WG III, Heidt RS Jr. Complete arthroscopic examination of the long head of the biceps tendon. Arthroscopy 2001;17:430–2.
28. Chen CH, Hsu KY, Chen WJ, et al. Incidence and severity of biceps long head tendon lesion in patients with complete rotator cuff tears. J Trauma 2005;58: 1189–93.
29. Gill HS, El Rassi G, Bahk MS, et al. Physical examination for partial tears of the biceps tendon. Am J Sports Med 2007;35:1334–40.
30. Boileau P, Ahrens PM, Hatzidakis AM. Entrapment of the long head of the biceps tendon: the hourglass biceps—a cause of pain and locking of the shoulder. J Shoulder Elbow Surg 2004;13:249–57.
31. Sharma P, Maffulli N. Biology of tendon injury: healing, modeling and remodeling. J Musculoskelet Neuronal Interact 2006;6:181–90.
32. Kibler WB, McMullen J. Scapular dyskinesis and its relation to shoulder pain. J Am Acad Orthop Surg 2003;11(2):142–51.
33. Lukasiewicz AC, McClure P, Michener L, et al. Comparison of 3-dimensional scapular position and orientation between subjects with and without shoulder impingement. J Orthop Sports Phys Ther 1999;29(10):574–83.
34. Solem-Bertoft E, Thuomas KA, Westerberg CE. The influence of scapular retraction and protraction on the width of the subacromial space. An MRI study. Clin Orthop Relat Res 1993;296:99–103.
35. Glousman R, Jobe F, Tibone J, et al. Dynamic electromyographic analysis of the throwing shoulder with glenohumeral instability. J Bone Joint Surg Am 1988;70: 220–6.
36. Guanche C, Knatt T, Solomonow M, et al. The synergistic action of the capsule and the shoulder muscles. Am J Sports Med 1995;23:301–6.
37. Synder SJ, Karzel RP, Del Pizzo W, et al. SLAP lesions of the shoulder. Arthroscopy 1990;5:274–9.
38. Andrews JR, Carson WG Jr, McLeod WD. Glenoid labrum tears related to the long head of the biceps. Am J Sports Med 1985;13:337–41.
39. Burkhart SS, Morgan CD. The peel-back mechanism: its role in producing and extending posterior type II SLAP lesions and its effect on SLAP repair rehabilitation. Arthroscopy 1998;14:637–40.
40. Gartsman GM, Taverna E. The incidence of glenohumeral joint abnormalities associated with full-thickness, reparable rotator cuff tears. Arthroscopy 1997; 13:450–5.
41. Burkhead WZ, Arcand MA, Zeman C, et al. The biceps tendon. In: Rockwood CA, Matsen FA, Wirth MA, et al, editors. The shoulder, vol. 2. Philadelphia: Saunders; 2004. p. 1059–119.
42. Curtis AS, Synder SJ. Evaluation and treatment of biceps tendon pathology. Orthop Clin North Am 1993;24:33–43.
43. Matsen F, Kirby R. Office evaluation and management of shoulder pain. Orthop Clin North Am 1982;13:45.
44. Neer CS II. Impingement lesions. Clin Orthop 1983;173:70–7.
45. Gilcreest EL, Albi P. Unusual lesions of muscles and tendons of the shoulder girdle and upper arm. Surg Gynecol Obstet 1939;68:903–17.
46. Yergason RM. Rupture of biceps. J Bone Joint Surg 1931;13:160.

47. O'Brien SJ, Pagnani MJ, Fealy S, et al. The active compression test: a new and effective test for diagnosing labral tears and acromioclavicular joint abnormality. Am J Sports Med 1998;25:610–3.

48. Ludington NA. Rupture of the long head of biceps flexor cubiti muscle. Am J Surg 1923;77:358–63.

49. Gerber C, Ganz R. Clinical assessment of instability of the shoulder with special reference to anterior and posterior drawer tests. J Bone Joint Surg Br 1984;66:551.

50. Rowe CR, Zarins B. Recurrent transient subluxation of the shoulder. J Bone Joint Surg Am 1981;63:863.

51. Ahrens PM, Boileau P. The long head of biceps and associated tendinopathy. J Bone Joint Surg Br 2007;89:1001–9.

52. Altchek D, Wolf B. Disorders of the biceps tendon. In: Krishnan S, Hawkins R, Warren R, editors. The shoulder and the overhead athlete. Philadelphia: Lippincott, Williams & Wilkins; 2004. p. 196–208.

53. Barber FA, Field LD, Ryu R. Biceps tendon and superior labrum injuries: decision-making. J Bone Joint Surg Am 2007;89:1844–55.

54. Kennedy JC, Willis RB. The effect of local steroid injections on tendons: a biomechanical and mcroscopic correlative study. Am J Sports Med 1976;4:11–21.

55. Neviaser RJ. Lesions of the biceps and tendinitis of the shoulder. Orthop Clin North Am 1980;11:343–8.

56. Maitland GD. Vertebral manipulation. 4th edition. Boston: Butterworth; 1977.

57. Wyke BD. The neurology of joints. Ann R Coll Surg Engl 1967;41(1):25–50.

58. Noyes FR, Mangine RE, Barber S. Early knee motion after open and arthroscopic anterior cruciate ligament reconstruction. Am J Sports Med 1987; 15(2):149–60.

59. Stackhouse SK, Eisennagel A, Eisennagel J, et al. Experimental pain inhibits infraspinatus activation during isometric external rotation. J Shoulder Elbow Surg 2013;22(4):478–84.

60. Langevin HM, Bouffard NA, Churchill DL, et al. Connective tissue fibroblast response to acupuncture: dose-dependent effect of bidirectional needle rotation. J Altern Complement Med 2007;13(3):355–60.

61. Kubo K, Yagima H, Takayama M, et al. Effects of acupuncture and heating on blood volume and oxygen saturation of human Achilles tendon in vivo. Eur J Appl Physiol 2010;109(3):545–50.

62. Shinbara H, Okubo M, Sumiya E, et al. Effects of manual acupuncture with sparrow pecking on muscle blood flow of normal and denervated hindlimb in rats. Acupunct Med 2008;26(3):149–59.

63. James SL, Ali K, Pocock C, et al. Ultrasound guided dry needling and autologous blood injection for patellar tendinosis. Br J Sports Med 2007;41(8): 518–21 [discussion: 522].

64. Lee JA, Jeong GH, Park HJ, et al. Acupuncture accelerates wound healing in burn-injured mice. Burns 2011;37(1):117–25.

65. Ballyns JJ, Shah JP, Hammond J, et al. Objective sonographic measures for characterizing myofascial trigger points associated with cervical pain. J Ultrasound Med 2011;30:1331–40.

66. Sikdar S, Shah JP, Gebreab T, et al. Novel applications of ultrasound technology to visualize and characterize myofascial trigger points and surrounding soft tissue. Arch Phys Med Rehabil 2009;90:1829–38.

67. Cook J, Purdham C. Is tendon pathology a continuum? A pathology based model to explain the clinical presentation of load induced tendinopathy. Br J Sports Med 2009;43(6):409–16.

68. Moseley GL. Teaching people about pain: why do we keep beating around the bush? Pain Manag 2012;2:1–3.
69. Arendt-Nielsen L, Castaldo M. MTPs are a peripheral source of nociception. Pain Med 2015;16(4):625–7.
70. Lucas KR, Rich PA, Polus BI. Muscle activation patterns in the scapular positioning muscles during loaded scapular plane elevation: the effects of latent myofascial trigger points. Clin Biomech 2010;25:765–80.
71. Sandberg M, Lundeberg T, Lindberg LG, et al. Effects of acupuncture on skin and muscle blood flow in healthy subjects. Eur J Appl Physiol 2003;90(1–2):114–9.
72. McShane JM, Nazarian LN, Harwood MI. Sonographically guided percutaneous needle tenotomy for treatment of common extensor tendinosis in the elbow. J Ultrasound Med 2006;25:1281–9.
73. Ridzki JR, Alder RS, Warren FR, et al. Contrast-enhanced ultrasound characterization of the vascularity of the rotator cuff tendon: age- and activity-related changes in the intact asymptomatic rotator cuff. J Shoulder Elbow Surg 2008;17(1 Suppl):96S–100S.
74. Suresh S, Ali K, Jones H, et al. Medial epicondylitis: is ultrasound guided autologous blood injection an effective treatment? Br J Sports Med 2006;40(11):935–9.
75. Kader D, Saxena A, Movin T, et al. Achilles tendinopathy: some aspects of basic science and clinical management. Br J Sports Med 2002;36:239–49.
76. Testa V, Maffulli N, Capasso G, et al. Percutaneous longitudinal tenotomy in chronic Achilles tendonitis. Bull Hosp Joint Dis 1996;54(4):241–4.
77. Hsieh JC, Tu CH, Chen FP, et al. Activation of the hypothalamus characterizes the acupuncture stimulation at the analgesic point in human: a positron emission tomography study. Neurosci Lett 2001;307(2):105–8.
78. Hui KK, Liu J, Makris N, et al. Acupuncture modulates the limbic system and subcortical gray structures of the human brain: evidence from fMRI studies in normal subjects. Hum Brain Mapp 2000;9(1):13–25.
79. Napadow V, Kettner N, Liu J, et al. Hypothalamus and amygdala response to acupuncture stimuli in Carpal Tunnel Syndrome. Pain 2007;130(3):254–66.
80. Napadow V, Makris N, Liu J, et al. Effects of electroacupuncture versus manual acupuncture on the human brain as measure by fMRI. Hum Brain Mapp 2005;24(3):193–205.
81. Biella G, Sotgiu ML, Pellegata G, et al. Acupuncture produces central activations in pain regions. Neuroimage 2001;14:60–6.
82. Wilk KE, Macrina LC, Fleisig GS, et al. Loss of internal rotation and the correlation to shoulder injuries in professional baseball pitchers. Am J Sports Med 2011;39:329–35.
83. Myers JB, Laudner KG, Pasquale MR, et al. Glenohumeral range of motion deficits and posterior shoulder tightness in throwers with pathologic internal impingement. Am J Sports Med 2006;34:385–91.
84. Wright RW, Steger-May K, Wasserlauf BL, et al. Elbow range of motion in professional baseball pitchers. Am J Sports Med 2006;34(2):190–3.
85. Borstad JD, Ludewig PM. Comparison of three stretches for the pectoralis minor muscle. J Shoulder Elbow Surg 2006;15(3):324–30.
86. Muraki T, Aoki M, Izumi T, et al. Lengthening of the pectoralis minor muscle during passive shoulder motions and stretching techniques: a cadaveric biomechanical study. Phys Ther 2009;89(4):333–41.
87. Kibler WB, Sciascia A, Dome D. Evaluation of apparent and absolute supraspinatus strength in patients with shoulder injury using the scapular retraction test. Am J Sports Med 2006;34(10):1643–7.

88. Seitz AL, McClure PW, Finucane S, et al. The scapular assistance test results in changes in scapular position and subacromial space but not rotator cuff strength in subacromial impingement. J Orthop Sports Phys Ther 2012;42(5):400–12.
89. Wilk KE, Arrigo CA, Andrews JR. Current concepts: the stabilization structures of the glenohumeral joint. J Orthop Sports Phys Ther 1997;25(6):364–79.
90. Wilk KE, Arrigo CA. An integrated approach to upper extremity exercises. Orthop Phys Ther Clin North Am 1992;1:337–60.
91. Poppen NK, Walker PS. Forces at the glenohumeral joint in abduction. Clin Orthop Relat Res 1978;(135):165–70.
92. Walker PS, Poppen NK. Biomechanics of the shoulder joint during abduction in the plane of the scapula [proceedings]. Bull Hosp Joint Dis 1977;38(2):107–11.
93. Lephart SM, Pincivero DM, Giraldo JL, et al. The role of proprioception in the management and rehabilitation of athletic injuries. Am J Sports Med 1997; 25(1):130–7.
94. Lephart SM, Warner JJ, Borsa PA, et al. Proprioception of the shoulder joint in healthy, unstable, and surgically repaired shoulders. J Shoulder Elbow Surg 1994;3(6):371–80.
95. Knott M, Voss DE. Proprioceptive neuromuscular facilitation: patterns and techniques. 2nd edition. New York: Hoeber; 1968.
96. Sullivan PE, Markos PD, Minor MAD. An integrated approach to therapeutic exercise: theory and clinical application. Reston (VA): Reston Publishing Company; 1982.
97. Wilk KE, Andrews JR, Arrigo C. Preventive and rehabilitative exercises for the shoulder and elbow. 6th edition. Birmingham (AL): American Sports Medicine Institute; 2001.
98. Wilk KE, Arrigo C, Andrews JR. Closed and open kinetic chain exercises for the upper extremity. J Sports Rehabil 1996;5:88–102.
99. Fleisig GS, Jameson GG, Cody KE, et al. Muscle activity during shoulder rehabilitation exercises. In: Proceedings of NACOB '98, The Third North American Congress on Biomechanics. Waterloo, Canada: 1998. p. 223–34.
100. Blackburn TA, McLeod WD, White B, et al. EMG analysis of posterior rotator cuff exercises. Athl Train 1990;25:40–5.
101. Decker MJ, Hintermeister RA, Faber KJ, et al. Serratus anterior muscle activity during selected rehabilitation exercises. Am J Sports Med 1992;7(6):784–91.
102. Hintermeister RA, Lange GW, Schultheis JM, et al. Electromyographic activity and applied load during shoulder rehabilitation exercises using elastic resistance. Am J Sports Med 1998;26:210–20.
103. Jobe FW, Tibone JE, Jobe CM, et al. The shoulder in sports. In: Rockwood CA Jr, Matsen FA III, editors. The shoulder. Philadelphia: WB Saunders; 1990. p. 961–90.
104. Pappas AM, Zawacki RM, McCarthy CF. Rehabilitation of the pitching shoulder. Am J Sports Med 1985;13(4):223–35.
105. Townsend H, Jobe FW, Pink M, et al. Electromyographic analysis of the glenohumeral muscles during a baseball rehabilitation program. Am J Sports Med 1991;19(3):264–72.
106. Moseley JB Jr, Jobe FW, Pink M, et al. EMG analysis of the scapular muscles during a shoulder rehabilitation program. Am J Sports Med 1992;29(2): 128–34.
107. Kibler WB. The role of the scapula in athletic shoulder function. Am J Sports Med 1998;26(2):325–7.
108. Kibler WB. Role of the scapula in overhead throwing motion. Contemp Orthop 1991;22:525–32.

109. Paine RM. The role of the scapula in the shoulder. In: Andrews JR, Wilk KE, editors. The athlete's shoulder. New York: Churchill Livingstone; 1994. p. 495–512.
110. Davies GJ, Dickoff-Hoffman S. Neuromuscular testing and rehabilitation of the shoulder complex. J Orthop Sports Phys Ther 1993;18(2):449–58.
111. Tucker WS, Armstrong CW, Gribble PA, et al. Scapular muscle activity in overhead athletes with symptoms of secondary shoulder impingement during closed chain exercises. Arch Phys Med Rehabil 2010;91(4):550–6.
112. Carpenter JE, Blasier RB, Pellizzon GG. The effects of muscle fatigue on shoulder joint position sense. Am J Sports Med 1998;26(2):262–5.
113. Tsai NT, McClure PW, Karduna AR. Effects of muscle fatigue on 3-dimensional scapular kinematics. Arch Phys Med Rehabil 2003;84:1000–5.
114. Wilk KE, Yenchak AJ, Arrigo CA, et al. The advanced throwers ten exercise program: a new exercise series for enhanced dynamic shoulder control in the overhead throwing athlete. Phys Sportsmed 2011;39(4):90–7.
115. Reinold MM, Wilk KE, Reed J, et al. Interval sport programs: guidelines for baseball, tennis, and golf. J Orthop Sports Phys Ther 2002;32(6):293–8.

Biceps Tenotomy Versus Tenodesis

Kushal V. Patel, MD[a],*, Jonathan Bravman, MD[b], Armando Vidal, MD[b],
Ashley Chrisman, PA-C[c], Eric McCarty, MD[b]

KEYWORDS

- Biceps tenodesis • Biceps tenotomy • Outcomes • Tenodesis technique
- Biceps surgical treatment

KEY POINTS

- An attempt at conservative treatment of long head biceps tendon, a common cause of anterior shoulder pain, should be undertaken initially. Conservative treatment includes physical therapy, activity modification, oral anti-inflammatory medication, and ultrasound-guided steroid injection.
- Surgical treatment of long head biceps tendon pain includes tenotomy or tenodesis. A myriad of different surgical techniques has been described for tenodesis and will likely to continue to evolve.
- Numerous studies have evaluated the outcomes between tenotomy and tenodesis; however, many of these studies have a low level of evidence and confounding factors. As a result, superiority of one procedure over the other has not been demonstrated.
- Tenotomy and tenodesis are both good surgical options for long head biceps pain. Patient and surgeon preference are likely the primary driving factors for choosing between the 2 procedures.

INTRODUCTION

The long head of the biceps, originating from the supraglenoid tubercle and superior glenoid labrum, is a common cause of anterior shoulder pain as the tendon

Disclosure Statement: No disclosures (K.V. Patel, A. Chrisman); royalties from Elsevier, research/education projects with Stryker, DePuy Synthes Mitek, Smith & Nephew, Biomet, Histogenics (E. McCarty); consultant: Ceterix, Stryker, Speakers bureau: Arhtrex (A. Vidal); consultant: DJO, Smith & Nephew (J. Bravman). Drs E. McCarty, A. Vidal, and J. Bravman have fellowship support from Stryker, Smith & Nephew, and Mitek.
a Baylor Scott and White Orthopaedics at Garland, 601 Clara Barton Boulevard, Plaza III, Suite 250, Garland, TX 75012, USA; b Department of Orthopaedics, Sports Medicine and Shoulder Surgery, CU Sports Medicine, University of Colorado Hospital, 311 Mapleton Avenue, Boulder, CO 80304, USA; c Department of Orthopaedics, CU Sports Medicine, University of Colorado Hospital, 311 Mapleton Avenue, Boulder, CO 80304, USA
* Corresponding author.
E-mail address: kvportho@gmail.com

Clin Sports Med 35 (2016) 93–111
http://dx.doi.org/10.1016/j.csm.2015.08.008
0278-5919/16/$ – see front matter © 2016 Elsevier Inc. All rights reserved.

traverses the glenohumeral joint coursing distally through the bicipital grove. The tendon pathologic condition can be classified into 3 basic categories: inflammatory, instability, and traumatic. Inflammatory lesions are the most common of these 3 causes.

PATHOLOGIC ENTITIES

Inflammation of the biceps tendon can involve the tendon itself or the surrounding bursa. Commonly, the 2 are present concomitantly. MR imaging without arthrogram contrast will often demonstrate excessive fluid within the bursa or flattening of the biceps tendon.[1] These features are most notable on the axial series. These inflammatory changes are commonly attributed to degenerative tendinopathy and overuse. Subacromial impingement can also lead to or be associated with bicipital tendinitis.[2–6] Gross visualization typically demonstrates an erythematous, misshaped tendon with accumulation of bursa, as shown in **Fig. 1**.

Second, instability of the tendon can lead to mechanical symptoms such as popping and clicking with range of motion, which patients typically ascribe to the anterior aspect of the shoulder. Pain can accompany the mechanical symptoms. In the presence of an unstable long head biceps tendon, the clinician should have a high suspicion of an associated subscapularis tendon tear. Physical examination findings of palpable or audible popping and clicking rather than the static MR images can help support the diagnosis. Subscapularis function should also be tested to rule out a tear. Furthermore, an unstable superior labral anterior posterior (SLAP) tear is another cause associated with biceps instability and pain.

Finally, the long head of the biceps is susceptible to traumatic injury. Typically, a complete rupture of the tendon is encountered. In these situations, pain resolves with time, and function is typically preserved. However, when trauma leads to partial tearing or splits within the tendon, pain necessitating treatment is common.

PREOPERATIVE MANAGEMENT

In patients who present with anterior shoulder pain, the long head of the biceps tendon must be included in the differential diagnosis. When pain and dysfunction have been

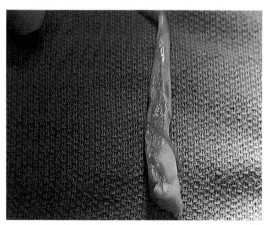

Fig. 1. Gross visualization of removed portion of the long head biceps tendon. Note the pathologic changes including tearing and tendinopathy.

attributed to the biceps, conservative treatment is commonly recommended initially. Treatment includes oral anti-inflammatories, activity modification, ultrasound-guided steroid injection, physical therapy, and modalities, including ultrasound, iontophoresis, electrical stimulation, and dry needling. Even in patients with mechanical symptoms and traumatic cause, conservative treatment is an option. Usually the mechanical symptoms persist; however, the associated pain and dysfunction can be alleviated. The authors prefer ultrasound-guided steroid injection to be both diagnostic and therapeutic. The use of ultrasound can confirm correct placement of the steroid within the bursa, as demonstrated in **Fig. 2**. In addition, ultrasound examination can provide information regarding flattening or tendinopathy as well as instability with dynamic evaluation (**Fig. 3**).

The authors' preferred conservative treatment pathway is illustrated in **Fig. 4**. In their practice, conservative treatment is trialed for 6 to 12 weeks. They prefer physical therapy and steroid injection as first-line treatments. When conservative treatment has failed, 2 common surgical options are available—biceps tenotomy and biceps tenodesis. **Box 1** lists common indications for surgical intervention.

PHYSICAL EXAMINATION

A systematic approach should be used when evaluating a patient for shoulder pain and includes visual inspection, palpation, range of motion testing both passive and active, strength testing, and special tests. Particularly, several physical examination findings can suggest long head biceps tendon pain (**Box 2**). Pain with palpation anteriorly along the bicipital groove, audible or palpable clicking or subluxation appreciated with shoulder range of motion, anterior shoulder pain with impingement testing, that is, Hawkins and Neer examination, pain with Speed and Yergason testing, anterior shoulder pain with O'Brien test, or pain with range of motion particularly with arm extension and external rotation can all suggest a pathologic long head biceps tendon. The examiner must keep in mind anterior shoulder pain may also be reproduced from lesions of the subscapularis; therefore, examination should include passive external rotation, lift off, belly press, and bear hug test of the subscapularis. Several studies have demonstrated the statistical reliability of these special tests in determining long head biceps pathologic condition. Unfortunately, many of these tests have mediocre sensitivities and specificities, as shown in **Table 1**.[7,8]

PREOPERATIVE PLANNING

Radiographs in every patient who presents with shoulder pain should be obtained. Typically, in the authors' practice, a shoulder series consisting of 4 images including a shoulder anteroposterior (AP), true shoulder AP (Grashey), axillary, and scapular-Y views is ordered. There are no radiographic findings suggesting long head biceps pathologic condition. However, findings such as acromion curvature on the scapular-Y or sclerosis of the greater tuberosity can signify the presence of subacromial impingement and rotator cuff pathologic condition. As stated above, the long head biceps tendon can be symptomatic in patients with subacromial impingement, and therefore, these radiographic findings can imply compression of long head biceps via subacromial impingement. Isolated long head biceps tendon pathologic condition is not common; rather, it is often present with rotator cuff disease and subacromial bursitis.

Unlike plain radiographs, MR imaging can demonstrate long head biceps tendinopathy, flattening, tearing, subluxation/dislocation, and synovial inflammation. MRI

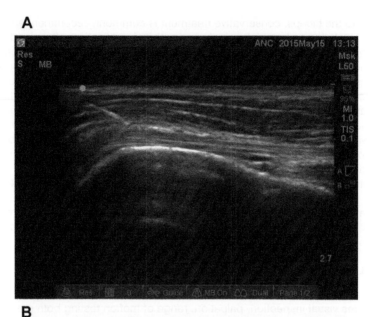

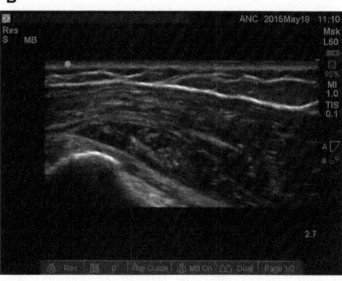

Fig. 2. (*A, B*) Ultrasound longitudinal figures of needle placement into the biceps tendon sheath and injection of steroid. (*B*) Steroid insufflation of the sheath. Green marker indicates ultrasound transducer orientation.

without intra-articular contrast is preferred because the contrast material can diffuse into the long head biceps tendon sheath and make it difficult to appreciate bursal inflammation. The axial T2 images provide the most information. Signal heterogeneity within the tendon suggests tendinopathy, and the amount of bursal fluid surrounding the tendon is noted, suggestive of inflammation. Furthermore, any dislocation or subluxation of the tendon out of the bicipital groove is easily identified (**Fig. 5**).

A

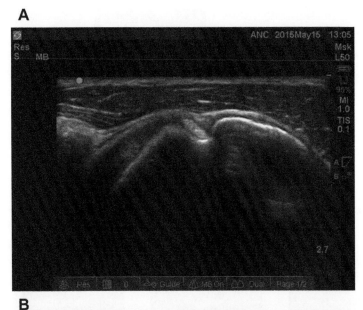

B

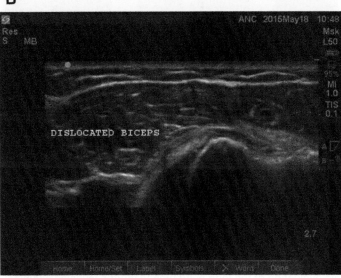

Fig. 3. (A, B) Axial ultrasound comparing a dislocated and reduced biceps tendon. Green marker indicates ultrasound transducer orientation.

TENODESIS VERSUS TENOTOMY

Several variables need to be considered when deciding between tenotomy and tenodesis (**Box 3**). They include age, functional demand postoperatively, cosmesis, body habitus, Workers' compensation status, and operative time. Some surgeons may elect to perform a tenotomy for its ease and decreased surgical time especially when multiple other procedures are planned, such as a rotator cuff repair and distal clavicle excision.

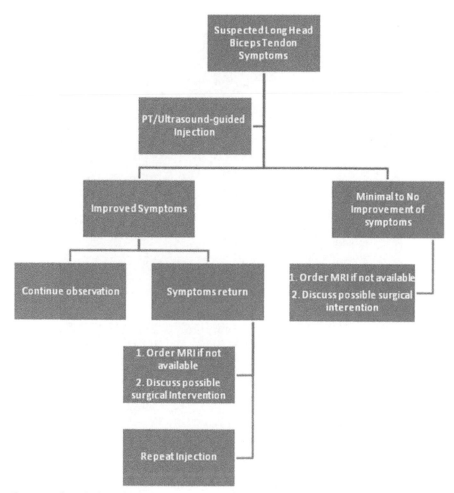

Fig. 4. Preferred algorithm of conservative treatment. PT, physical therapy.

ARTHROSCOPIC EVALUATION OF THE LONG HEAD BICEPS TENDON

Arthroscopic evaluation of the long head biceps tendon involves examination of the tendon itself for any fraying, tearing, erythema, and vascular injection. The bicipital groove portion is brought into the joint and visualized as well; this can easily be done by placing traction on the tendon with a probe. The authors prefer to place the probe superior to the tendon and pull the tendon anterior and inferior so as not to disrupt visualization. Furthermore, the superior labrum is examined for tear and instability of the biceps anchor via either re-creation of the peel back mechanism or manual traction with a probe. Finally, evaluation of the medial sling (biceps pulley), including the coracohumeral and superior glenohumeral ligament, is visualized at the upper border of the subscapularis (**Fig. 6**). With unstable tendons, there will be disruption of this medial sling and likely an associated subscapularis tear.

Box 1
Indications for surgical intervention
Long head biceps tendon injury/tear
Instability
Tenosynovitis/bursitis
Bicipital groove pain/positive clinical examination
Failed conservative treatment
SLAP tear
Combined subscapularis tear and medial biceps tendon subluxation

SURGICAL OPTIONS

Surgical options for the treatment of long head biceps tendon include tenotomy or tenodesis (**Table 2**). Tenotomy is performed arthroscopically with one fundamental technique. Recently, however, a looped arthroscopic tenotomy has been described.[9] A myriad of different surgical techniques has been described for tenodesis, including arthroscopic and open techniques.

SURGICAL TECHNIQUES
Arthroscopic Biceps Tenotomy

An arthroscopic biceps tenotomy is a rather quick and technically simple procedure. The authors prefer to do this in the beach chair position with the arm in neutral rotation with 90° of elbow flexion, with the arm in an arm holder. Viewing from the standard posterior portal and having developed an anterior superior portal, an arthroscopic biter or Metzenbaum scissors is used to cut the long head tendon. The tendon is transected at its origin from the superior labrum. The tendon tends to retract into the bicipital groove. Commonly, an arthroscopic resector is necessary to trim the remaining intra-articular stump to prevent any future mechanical symptoms and pain. The arthroscopic resector is also used to suction any tendon pieces in the joint and smooth the superior labrum. Care is taken not to disrupt the superior glenohumeral ligament when attending to the superior labrum. The tenotomy is performed after a diagnostic evaluation has been completed of the joint.

Arthroscopic Looped Tenotomy

The technique article was described by Goubier and colleagues.[9] In this technique, the intra-articular biceps tendon is looped within itself after being tenotomized from the

Box 2
Long head biceps physical examination tests
Palpation of the bicipital groove
Speed test
Yergason test
O'Brien test
Anterior shoulder pain with arm extension

Table 1
Statistical reliability of physical examination test for long head biceps pathologic condition

Test	Sensitivity	Specificity	Positive Predictive Value	Negative Predictive Value
Speed	0.54	0.81	0.56	0.79
Yergason	0.41	0.79	0.48	0.74
O'Brien	0.38	0.61	0.31	0.67

Data from Holtby R, Razmjou H. Accuracy of the Speed's and Yergason's tests in detecting biceps pathology and SLAP lesions: comparison with arthroscopic findings. Arthroscopy 2004;20(3): 231–6; and Bennett WF. Specificity of the Speed's test: arthroscopic technique for evaluating the biceps tendon at the level of the bicipital groove. Arthroscopy 1998;14(8):789–96.

superior labrum. Theoretically, the looped tendon prevents retraction into the bicipital groove; thereby avoiding a Popeye deformity and muscle cramps associated with the traditional long head biceps tenotomy. Clinical outcomes have not been studied with this technique, however.

Tenodesis

Several different techniques of tenodesis have been described. When performing a tenodesis, the surgeon should consider fixation method (ie interference screw, suture anchor, or sutureless anchor), position relative to the pectoralis major muscle tendon (suprapectoral vs subpectoral), intraosseous or extraosseous fixation, and arthroscopic or open technique. In the authors' practice, they perform a mini-open subpectoral tenodesis with a suture anchor. They think this method is optimal because it removes any pathologic extra-articular lesions and minimizes residual postoperative anterior shoulder pain by ensuring the tendon and synovium are removed from the bicipital groove, which the authors think is a pain generator. Moon and colleagues[10] demonstrated that 80% of tendons had degenerative changes beyond 5.6 cm from the glenoid tubercle under histologic evaluation. Therefore, a subpectoral tenodesis potentially eliminates any remaining painful tendon and bursa. In the authors' practice, the biceps tenodesis is performed before arthroscopy of the shoulder in most of their cases. The authors perform tenodesis before arthroscopy because the decision to perform tenodesis is typically determined preoperatively and typically does not change based on intraoperative findings; this is because they have found many of the true lesions of the biceps tendon are ultimately found to be hidden and not

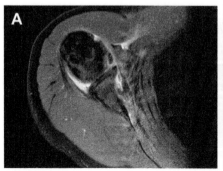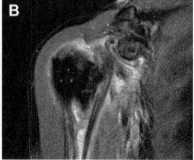

Fig. 5. (*A*, *B*) T2 axial and coronal MRI slices demonstrating a dislocated long head biceps tendon.

| **Box 3** |
| **Tenotomy or tenodesis: factors to consider** |
| Age |
| Functional activity and demand |
| Cosmetic concern |
| Body habitus |
| Workers' compensation status |
| Operating room time/number of concomitant surgical procedures |
| Patient compliance with postoperative restrictions |

thoroughly appreciated until the nonvisualized portion has been removed from beneath the transverse humeral ligament.[10] However, if a decision is necessary intraoperatively, the intra-articular portion is visualized during the diagnostic evaluation, and the tendon is assessed as described above (**Fig. 7**).

Mini-Open Subpectoral Biceps Tenodesis

- The arm is positioned in slight external rotation and abduction. The elbow is positioned at 90° of flexion (**Fig. 8**A).
- The incision is in the axillary crease with the superior third over the inferior margin of the pectoralis major muscle. The arm is adducted before marking the skin incision to see if any axillary creases can be used for the incision (**Fig. 8**B).
- Blunt dissection is carried down to the fascia and then under the pectoralis major muscle and tendon. Once under the inferior edge, blunt dissection is carried superiorly and laterally over the lateral margin of the humerus (**Fig. 8**C).
- A small Hohmann retractor is then placed on the lateral margin of the humerus, taking care not to retract the long head biceps tendon itself. The long and short heads of the biceps are then visualized. The short head of the biceps is retracted with another small Hohmann or blunt retractor. Care should be taken to avoid aggressive retraction on the short head to prevent any iatrogenic injury to the

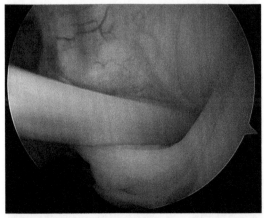

Fig. 6. The medial sling and the biceps tendon as it enters the bicipital groove. The patient is in a lateral decubitus position.

Table 2 Surgical options	
Tenotomy	**Tenodesis**
Arthroscopic tenotomy	Arthroscopic soft tissue tenodesis
Arthroscopic looped tenotomy	Arthroscopic suture anchor tenodesis
	Arthroscopic knotless anchor tenodesis
	Mini-open suture anchor subpectoral tenodesis
	Min-open interference screw subpectoral tenodesis
	Mini-open key hole tenodesis
	Mini-open bone tunnel tenodesis

musculocutaneous nerve. Commonly, there is a bursal layer over the long head biceps tendon. This bursal layer is easily removed by sweeping a lap sponge along the tendon to bluntly separate the bursa and synovium from the tendon (**Fig. 8**D).

- Once the long head biceps tendon is visualized, the musculotendinous junction is identified. The anticipated tenodesis site is 1 to 2 cm from the musculotendinous junction. The tendon is retracted laterally; any bursal tissue and proliferation are excised, and then the bicipital groove is curetted at the level of tenodesis.
- A suture anchor is placed in the curetted area, and sutures are placed into the tendon in a lasso fashion (**Fig. 8**E).
- A hemostat is positioned proximal to the tenodesis, and the tendon is cut between the 2 (**Fig. 8**F).
- The biceps is then cut intra-articularly, and the stump is removed from the axillary incision. In cutting the tendon after the tenodesis, the authors hope to maintain the length tension relationship of the tendon. Furthermore, they use an all suture-based anchor that requires a 2.9-mm drill hole; thus, minimizing the chance of an iatrogenic humerus fracture. An interference screw can also be used instead of a suture anchor.
- The axillary incision, once healed, is very nicely hidden (**Fig. 8**G, H).

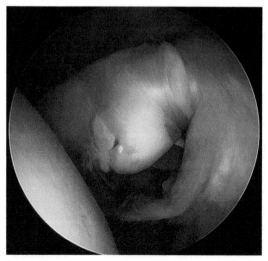

Fig. 7. Tear of the biceps tendon.

Several other techniques have been described, including the arthroscopic percutaneous intra-articular transtendon technique,[11] keyhole technique,[12] bone tunnel technique,[13] and arthroscopic interference screw technique.[14] The number of described techniques continues to evolve. The technique chosen by the surgeon is largely based on experience and comfort. Recent evaluation of the trend in biceps tenodesis demonstrated an increasing number of procedures for open and arthroscopic biceps tenodesis from 2008 to 2011 with the arthroscopic procedures outpacing the open procedures.[15] This study also illustrated a significant increase in the number of biceps tenodesis performed in patients aged 60 to 69 potentially questioning the general recommendations of performing a tenotomy in older, less active patients. In addition, the study noted an increased number of tenodesis in patients aged 20 to 29 and possibly attributed this to the treatment of SLAP tears or failed SLAP tears.[15]

RESULTS AND CLINICAL OUTCOMES

Numerous studies have evaluated the outcomes after tenodesis and tenotomy. Despite this, there has been a failure to demonstrate superiority of one technique over the other secondary to several factors. First, many of the studies involved patients undergoing either a tenotomy or a tenodesis with a concomitant surgical intervention. Comparison between the 2 procedures is difficult secondary to the potential influence of other shoulder pathologic condition.[2–6] Second, many of the studies are retrospective, with a lack of high-level evidence, and the variability of the biceps tenodesis technique makes it difficult to truly assess tenodesis as a whole, although several conclusions can still be drawn based on the currently available literature (**Table 3**).

COSMETIC DEFORMITY

Variable among patients, the importance of cosmesis can influence decision-making between biceps tenodesis versus biceps tenotomy. Releasing the proximal origin of the long head biceps tendon from the superior labrum and supraglenoid tubercle impacts the length tension relationship of the biceps and potentially creates a deformity commonly referred to as the "Popeye" deformity (**Fig. 9**). In a review article by Hsu and colleagues,[16] 41% and 25% of patients had a Popeye deformity after a biceps tenotomy and tenodesis, respectively. The reported odds ratio was 2.15 for a deformity with biceps tenotomy. Interestingly, 25% of patients who underwent biceps tenodesis had a deformity; this may be attributed to failure of the tenodesis or to inappropriate tensioning of the long head tendon during tenodesis. In the authors' practice, they commonly tenodese the tendon before releasing the intra-articular portion to help prevent this and maintain the length tension relationship of the muscle belly, although this has not yet been systematically validated. Furthermore, the amount of subcutaneous tissue present should be considered as well. The deformity may not be as appreciable in patients with a greater amount of subcutaneous adipose tissue, and second, a tenodesis may be more technically challenging in these patients. Patients should be counseled that a Popeye deformity may be present with either technique; however, in the authors' experience, they have seen significantly lower rates of a Popeye deformity after tenodesis than reported above. Men potentially have a higher incidence of Popeye deformity than women after tenotomy.[17] The higher incidence of Popeye deformity with tenotomy has been demonstrated and corroborated in multiple other studies.[4,5,18–22]

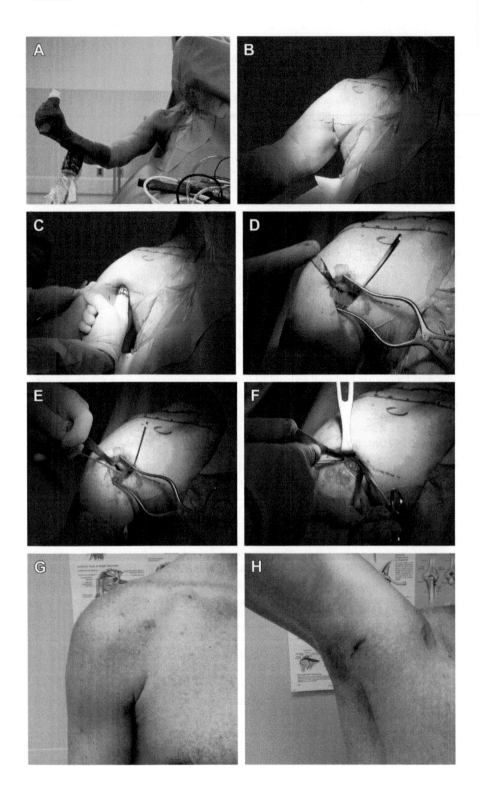

SUBJECTIVE OUTCOMES

No clinically statistical difference has been demonstrated between tenotomy and tenodesis.[3,6,23] A systematic review by Frost and colleagues[24] demonstrated a nonsuperiority of one technique over the other. Forty percent to 100% in the tenodesis group and 65% to 100% in the tenotomy group had good to excellent outcomes. Furthermore, failure rates were reported as 5% to 48% and 13% to 35% in the tenodesis and tenotomy group, respectively.[24] These findings have been supported by other studies, demonstrating 84% excellent, 11% fair, and 5% poor outcomes after tenotomy.[17,25]

When considering outcome scores, several studies have corroborated similar results among patients who underwent a tenotomy and tenodesis. A systematic review evaluated Constant and UCLA (University of California Los Angeles) scores in the 2 groups. Constant scores were reported to average 66.9 and 76.1 in patients who underwent tenotomy and tenodesis, respectively[4,16,25,26]; UCLA scores averaged 33 for tenotomy and 28 for tenodesis.[16,17,27] The subjective findings of the studies were not statistically significant. Koh and colleagues[18] prospectively evaluated patients who underwent rotator cuff repair and either biceps tenodesis or tenotomy and demonstrated no difference in ASES (American Shoulder and Elbow Surgeons) score and Constant score. Even at 2 years after surgical intervention, no difference has been documented.[23,24] Despite the lack of statistical difference in outcomes, there has been documented greater improvement in Constant scores with tenodesis than with tenotomy.[4,18–21] However, evaluation of patient satisfaction has demonstrated similar findings among the 2 procedures[4,18–20] despite potentially greater improvement in Constant scores with tenodesis.

When examining either arthroscopic suprapectoral or open subpectoral tenodesis, no difference in ASES scores, patient satisfaction, or return to athletic activity was found when patients with concomitant rotator cuff or labral repair were excluded.[28] The lack of clinical difference between suprapectoral and subpectoral tenodesis has been demonstrated in other studies with ASES scores of 89 in open subpectoral tenodesis and 78 in arthroscopic suprapectoral tenodesis.[29–31] The presence of a rotator cuff lesion and its influence on outcomes have also been studied. Mazzocca and colleagues [29] demonstrated that postoperative ASES scores were statistically better in patients without concomitant rotator cuff lesion in comparison to those who underwent open subpectoral tenodesis with a rotator cuff lesion.

Fatigue/cramping of the biceps muscle has also been a topic of evaluation. Fatigue discomfort has been reported after biceps tenotomy, particularly in younger patients. Kelly and colleagues[17] reported fatigue discomfort in 64%, 42%, and 0% in patients younger than 40, 40 to 60, and older than 60, respectively, who underwent tenotomy. Multiple other studies have supported higher incidence of muscle cramping and pain with tenotomy.[4,18–20]

Fig. 8. (*A*) The arm is positioned in neutral to slight external rotation and flexion. (*B*) An incision is marked in line with an axillary crease with the upper third at the inferior border of the pectoralis major muscle. (*C*) After incision through the fascia, blunt dissection is carried out under the pectoralis major muscle out laterally. (*D*) Exposure of the tendon is obtained by placing a Hohmann retractor laterally over the humerus. A self-retaining retractor and another retractor medially can also help. (*E*) The sutures from the placed anchor are then stitched into the tendon. (*F*) The tendon is cut proximal the tenodesis site. (*G*) Six weeks postoperatively demonstrating good cosmetic outcome with the scar only visualized with the arm in abduction (*H*).

Table 3
Tenotomy versus tenodesis

	Tenotomy	Tenodesis
Pros	Technically easier	Lower incidence Popeye deformity
	Fewer postoperative restrictions	Maintenance of length-tension relationship
	Quicker recovery	Possibly improved supination strength
	Shorter operative time	—
Cons	Higher incidence Popeye deformity	More postoperative restrictions
	Muscle cramping/fatigue	Longer recovery
	—	Longer operative time

RESIDUAL POSTOPERATIVE BICIPITAL SHOULDER PAIN

When considering tenotomy or tenodesis and residual postoperative bicipital pain, a review article by Hsu and colleagues[16] demonstrated a higher odds ratios (1.5) and relative risk (1.4) of postoperative bicipital pain in the tenodesis group with 17% versus 24% of patients in the tenotomy and tenodesis group, respectively, having postoperative bicipital pain. When examining suprapectoral and subpectoral tenodesis techniques, many studies have favored improved postoperative resolution of bicipital pain with the subpectoral technique. Two of 5 patients in the suprapectoral group compared with zero patients in the subpectoral group demonstrated residual anterior shoulder tenderness in the study by Lutton and colleagues.[31] Mazzocca and colleagues[29] noted complete resolution of bicipital groove pain in patients who underwent open subpectoral tenodesis with an interference screw at an average of 29 months. Thus, subpectoral tenodesis may be more reliable in eliminating anterior shoulder pain from the long head biceps tendon. Pathologic lesions of the tendon,

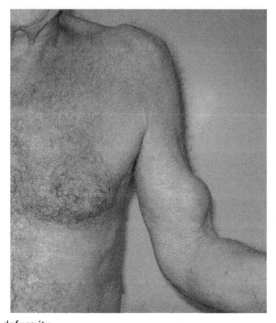

Fig. 9. A Popeye deformity.

including tears and tenosynovitis extending into the distal aspect of the bicipital groove, have been shown.[10] As a result, a suprapectoral tenodesis can potentially fail to remove the pain-generating portion of the tendon or etiologic pathologic condition.[31–34]

OBJECTIVE OUTCOMES

Postoperative flexion and supination strength have been examined after tenotomy and tenodesis; the results have been variable. Overall, there has been no high level of evidence to support improved objective results of one technique over the other. No difference in elbow flexion strength,[2,17,18,23,35] flexion endurance,[23] and supination strength[23,35] has been demonstrated. On the other hand, decreased supination and flexion strength with tenotomy have been demonstrated in certain populations.[17,35] When examining range of motion postoperatively, no difference between the 2 in terms of forward flexion, external rotation, and internal rotation[4,5,20] has been concluded.

REVISION RATES

Revision rates may potentially be improved with a mini-open subpectoral tenodesis compared with suprapectoral tenodesis. Sanders and colleagues[34] demonstrated a revision rate of 20.6% in proximal tenodesis or tenotomy compared with a rate of 7.7% in a distal tenodesis. Friedman and colleagues[36] reported a revision rate of 12% compared with 2.7% after 2 years in patients who underwent tenodesis proximal and distal to the groove, respectively.

COMPLICATIONS

In one study, complication rates over a 3-year period in patients after subpectoral biceps tenodesis with an interference screw were relatively low with 0.57% persistent bicipital pain, 0.57% loss of fixation, 0.28% deep postoperative wound infection, and 0.28% musculocutaneous neuropathy.[37] Gombera and colleagues[28] demonstrated no complications with an all-arthroscopic tenodesis group compared with 2 complications in the open subpectoral tenodesis of a superficial wound infection and a brachial plexopathy that resolved 5 months postoperatively. Other concerns of tenodesis are fracture-, hematoma-, and implant-related reaction, continued discomfort in the subpectoral triangle, and a 2% failure rate of fixation.[29] The concern for iatrogenic humerus fracture with a tenodesis is valid, and several studies have highlighted key technical points. In mini-open subpectoral tenodesis with an interference screw, lateral eccentric drill hole placement for an 8-mm screw significantly reduced humeral strength.[38] Second, the location of a suprapectoral tenodesis may potentially lower the risk of iatrogenic humeral fracture because the humeral width is wider than the subpectoral site.

Some surgeons favor tenotomy or a suprapectoral tenodesis because there is concern over the proximity of brachial plexus to the subpectoral tenodesis site; this may place the neurovascular structures at risk, particularly with deep dissection and retraction of the short head of the biceps.[37,39,40] Dickens and colleagues[41] in a cadaveric study demonstrated the risk of injury to the musculocutaneous nerve, radial nerve, and deep brachial artery with medial retraction in an open technique. The study also noted that external rotation increases the distance from the tenodesis site to the musculocutaneous nerve compared with internal rotation of the arm. Jarrett and colleagues[42] illustrated that the musculocutaneous nerve averaged 2.6 cm from the long head biceps musculotendinous junction, and the anterior humeral circumflex vessels averaged 4.6 cm from the musculotendinous junction. However, arthroscopic suprapectoral tenodesis is not completely void of potential nerve injury. A cadaveric study demonstrated that a low anterolateral portal for tenodesis touched a small distal axillary nerve branch in almost half the shoulders.[43]

BIOMECHANICAL EVALUATION

Numerous studies have examined the biomechanical differences of the various tenodesis techniques. To the authors' knowledge, only one study has biomechanically compared tenotomy with tenodesis. Wolf and colleagues[44] examined load to failure (defined as migration of the biceps stump distal to the bicipital groove) in a cadaveric model and found significantly higher load to failure with tenodesis: 110.7 N for tenotomy and 310.8 N for tenodesis. The remaining studies examined only the different tenodesis techniques. Sampatacos and colleagues[45] examined all arthroscopic biceps tenodesis with either an interference screw or an intraosseous suture fixation. The intraosseous suture fixation demonstrated a statistically greater load to failure, although the interference screw fixation had significant greater stiffness with cyclic loading. Furthermore, biomechanical evaluation of 4 tenodesis techniques (open subpectoral bone tunnel, arthroscopic interference screw, open subpectoral interference screw, and arthroscopic suture anchor) demonstrated no statistically significant difference in ultimate failure strength. The open subpectoral bone tunnel technique showed the highest displacement with cyclic loading and the least displacement was found in open interference screw fixation; however, no statistical difference between the open and arthroscopic techniques was noted.[46] Superior fixation strength with interference screw tenodesis has been supported by Ozalay and colleagues,[47] who demonstrated maximum load to failure with interference screw of 243.3 ± 72.4 N compared with 229.2 ± 44.1 N for tunnel technique, 129.0 ± 16.6 N for anchor technique, and 101.7 ± 27.9 N for keyhole technique. The study involved an ovine animal model and was performed in a single load-to-failure evaluation. Suture anchor fixation has become more popular. As a result, when comparing interference screw tenodesis and suture anchor fixation, Richards and Burkhart[48] demonstrated a statistically greater pullout strength for interference screw (233.5 ± 55.5 N) than double suture anchor fixation (135.5 ± 37.8 N) in a cadaveric biomechanical study. Whether this difference is clinically significant especially with the postoperative restrictions for a tenodesis is questionable.

POSTOPERATIVE REHABILITATION PROTOCOL

In patients with isolated biceps tenotomy, the arm is placed in a sling postoperatively for approximately 1 week for comfort, with a focus on early active and passive range of motion. As pain subsides, return to activity is allowed. As for biceps tenodesis, a sling is used for 4 weeks with no active elbow flexion and supination. Passive range of motion is allowed. At 4 weeks, the sling is removed, and active range of motion is started. Strengthening begins at 6 weeks. The effect on outcomes of various postoperative protocols has not been systematically studied to the authors' knowledge at this point in time.

SUMMARY

Long head biceps tendon pathologic condition is a common source of anterior shoulder pain. When conservative treatment fails, both tenotomy and tenodesis are reliable surgical options with good surgical outcomes. Higher-powered and higher level of evidence studies are necessary to truly evaluate the statistical and clinical difference between the 2 different options. Several factors influence the decision process on which technique to use. Surgeons should be familiar with the 2 techniques and their outcomes because either option can be appropriate for different patients.

REFERENCES

1. Dubrow SA, Streit JJ, Shishani Y, et al. Diagnostic accuracy in detecting tears in the proximal biceps tendon using standard nonenhancing shoulder MRI. Open Access J Sports Med 2014;5:81–7.
2. Wittstein J, Queen R, Abbey A, et al. Isokinetic testing of biceps strength and endurance in dominant versus nondominant upper extremities. J Shoulder Elbow Surg 2010;19(6):874–7.
3. Edwards TB, Walch G, Sirveaux F, et al. Repair of tears of the subscapularis. J Bone Joint Surg Am 2005;87(4):725–30.
4. Boileau P, Baqué F, Valerio L, et al. Isolated arthroscopic biceps tenotomy or tenodesis improves symptoms in patients with massive irreparable rotator cuff tears. J Bone Joint Surg Am 2007;89(4):747–57.
5. Franceschi F, Longo UG, Ruzzini L, et al. No advantages in repairing a type II superior labrum anterior and posterior (SLAP) lesion when associated with rotator cuff repair in patients over age 50: a randomized controlled trial. Am J Sports Med 2008;36(2):247–53.
6. Osbahr DC, Diamond AB, Speer KP. The cosmetic appearance of the biceps muscle after long-head tenotomy versus tenodesis. Arthroscopy 2002;18(5): 483–7.
7. Holtby R, Razmjou H. Accuracy of the Speed's and Yergason's tests in detecting biceps pathology and SLAP lesions: comparison with arthroscopic findings. Arthroscopy 2004;20(3):231–6.
8. Bennett WF. Specificity of the Speed's test: arthroscopic technique for evaluating the biceps tendon at the level of the bicipital groove. Arthroscopy 1998;14(8): 789–96.
9. Goubier JN, Bihel T, Dubois E, et al. Loop biceps tenotomy: an arthroscopic technique for long head of biceps tenotomy. Arthrosc Tech 2014;3(4):e427–30.
10. Moon SC, Cho NS, Rhee YG. Analysis of "hidden lesions" of the extra-articular biceps after subpectoral biceps tenodesis: the subpectoral portion as the optimal tenodesis site. Am J Sports Med 2015;43(1):63–8.
11. Sekiya JK, Elkousy HA, Rodosky MW. Arthroscopic biceps tenodesis using the percutaneous intra-articular transtendon technique. Arthroscopy 2003;19(10): 1137–41.
12. Froimson AI, O I. Keyhole tenodesis of biceps origin at the shoulder. Clin Orthop Relat Res 1975;(112):245–9.
13. Post M, Benca P. Primary tendinitis of the long head of the biceps. Clin Orthop Relat Res 1989;(246):117–25.
14. Lo IK, Burkhart SS. Arthroscopic biceps tenodesis using a bioabsorbable interference screw. Arthroscopy 2004;20(1):85–95.
15. Werner BC, Brockmeier SF, Gwathmey FW. Trends in long head biceps tenodesis. Am J Sports Med 2015;43(3):570–8.
16. Hsu AR, Ghodadra NS, Provencher MT, et al. Biceps tenotomy versus tenodesis: a review of clinical outcomes and biomechanical results. J Shoulder Elbow Surg 2011;20(2):326–32.

17. Kelly AM, Drakos MC, Fealy S, et al. Arthroscopic release of the long head of the biceps tendon: functional outcome and clinical results. Am J Sports Med 2005; 33(2):208–13.

18. Koh KH, Ahn JH, Kim SM, et al. Treatment of biceps tendon lesions in the setting of rotator cuff tears: prospective cohort study of tenotomy versus tenodesis. Am J Sports Med 2010;38(8):1584–90.

19. Zhang Q, Zhou J, Ge H, et al. Tenotomy or tenodesis for long head biceps lesions in shoulders with reparable rotator cuff tears: a prospective randomised trial. Knee Surg Sports Traumatol Arthrosc 2015;23(2):464–9.

20. Cho NS, Cha SW, Rhee YG. Funnel tenotomy versus intracuff tenodesis for lesions of the long head of the biceps tendon associated with rotator cuff tears. Am J Sports Med 2014;42(5):1161–8.

21. De Carli A, Vadalà A, Zanzotto E, et al. Reparable rotator cuff tears with concomitant long-head biceps lesions: tenotomy or tenotomy/tenodesis? Knee Surg Sports Traumatol Arthrosc 2012;20(12):2553–8.

22. Delle Rose G, Borroni M, Silvestro A, et al. The long head of biceps as a source of pain in active population: tenotomy or tenodesis? A comparison of 2 case series with isolated lesions. Musculoskelet Surg 2012;96(Suppl 1):S47–52.

23. Wittstein JR, Queen R, Abbey A, et al. Isokinetic strength, endurance, and subjective outcomes after biceps tenotomy versus tenodesis: a postoperative study. Am J Sports Med 2011;39(4):857–65.

24. Frost A, Zafar MS, Maffulli N. Tenotomy versus tenodesis in the management of pathologic lesions of the tendon of the long head of the biceps brachii. Am J Sports Med 2009;37(4):828–33.

25. Boileau P, Krishnan SG, Coste JS, et al. Arthroscopic biceps tenodesis: a new technique using bioabsorbable interference screw fixation. Arthroscopy 2002; 18(9):1002–12.

26. Walch G, Edwards TB, Boulahia A, et al. Arthroscopic tenotomy of the long head of the biceps in the treatment of rotator cuff tears: clinical and radiographic results of 307 cases. J Shoulder Elbow Surg 2005;14(3):238–46.

27. Checchia SL, Doneux PS, Miyazaki AN, et al. Biceps tenodesis associated with arthroscopic repair of rotator cuff tears. J Shoulder Elbow Surg 2005;14(2):138–44.

28. Gombera MM, Kahlenberg CA, Nair R, et al. All-arthroscopic suprapectoral versus open subpectoral tenodesis of the long head of the biceps brachii. Am J Sports Med 2015;43(5):1077–83.

29. Mazzocca AD, Cote MP, Arciero CL, et al. Clinical outcomes after subpectoral biceps tenodesis with an interference screw. Am J Sports Med 2008;36(10): 1922–9.

30. Werner BC, Evans CL, Holzgrefe RE, et al. Arthroscopic suprapectoral and open subpectoral biceps tenodesis: a comparison of minimum 2-year clinical outcomes. Am J Sports Med 2014;42(11):2583–90.

31. Lutton DM, Gruson KI, Harrison AK, et al. Where to tenodese the biceps: proximal or distal? Clin Orthop Relat Res 2011;469(4):1050–5.

32. Johannsen AM, Macalena JA, Carson EW, et al. Anatomic and radiographic comparison of arthroscopic suprapectoral and open subpectoral biceps tenodesis sites. Am J Sports Med 2013;41(12):2919–24.

33. Provencher MT, LeClere LE, Romeo AA. Subpectoral biceps tenodesis. Sports Med Arthrosc 2008;16(3):170–6.

34. Sanders B, Lavery KP, Pennington S, et al. Clinical success of biceps tenodesis with and without release of the transverse humeral ligament. J Shoulder Elbow Surg 2012;21(1):66–71.

35. Shank JR, Singleton SB, Braun S, et al. A comparison of forearm supination and elbow flexion strength in patients with long head of the biceps tenotomy or tenodesis. Arthroscopy 2011;27(1):9–16.
36. Friedman DJ, Dunn JC, Higgins LD, et al. Proximal biceps tendon: injuries and management. Sports Med Arthrosc 2008;16(3):162–9.
37. Nho SJ, Reiff SN, Verma NN, et al. Complications associated with subpectoral biceps tenodesis: low rates of incidence following surgery. J Shoulder Elbow Surg 2010;19(5):764–8.
38. Euler SA, Smith SD, Williams BT, et al. Biomechanical analysis of subpectoral biceps tenodesis: effect of screw malpositioning on proximal humeral strength. Am J Sports Med 2015;43(1):69–74.
39. Rhee PC, Spinner RJ, Bishop AT, et al. Iatrogenic brachial plexus injuries associated with open subpectoral biceps tenodesis: a report of 4 cases. Am J Sports Med 2013;41(9):2048–53.
40. Ma H, Van Heest A, Glisson C, et al. Musculocutaneous nerve entrapment: an unusual complication after biceps tenodesis. Am J Sports Med 2009;37(12): 2467–9.
41. Dickens JF, Kilcoyne KG, Tintle SM, et al. Subpectoral biceps tenodesis: an anatomic study and evaluation of at-risk structures. Am J Sports Med 2012; 40(10):2337–41.
42. Jarrett CD, McClelland WB Jr, Xerogeanes JW. Minimally invasive proximal biceps tenodesis: an anatomical study for optimal placement and safe surgical technique. J Shoulder Elbow Surg 2011;20(3):477–80.
43. Knudsen ML, Hibbard JC, Nuckley DJ, et al. The low-anterolateral portal for arthroscopic biceps tenodesis: description of technique and cadaveric study. Knee Surg Sports Traumatol Arthrosc 2014;22(2):462–6.
44. Wolf RS, Zheng N, Weichel D. Long head biceps tenotomy versus tenodesis: a cadaveric biomechanical analysis. Arthroscopy 2005;21(2):182–5.
45. Sampatacos N, Getelman MH, Henninger HB. Biomechanical comparison of two techniques for arthroscopic suprapectoral biceps tenodesis: interference screw versus implant-free intraosseous tendon fixation. J Shoulder Elbow Surg 2014; 23(11):1731–9.
46. Mazzocca AD, Bicos J, Santangelo S, et al. The biomechanical evaluation of four fixation techniques for proximal biceps tenodesis. Arthroscopy 2005;21(11): 1296–306.
47. Ozalay M, Akpinar S, Karaeminogullari O, et al. Mechanical strength of four different biceps tenodesis techniques. Arthroscopy 2005;21(8):992–8.
48. Richards DP, Burkhart SS. A biomechanical analysis of two biceps tenodesis fixation techniques. Arthroscopy 2005;21(7):861–6.

Arthroscopic Surgical Techniques for the Management of Proximal Biceps Injuries

Brian C. Werner, MD[a], Russell E. Holzgrefe, BS, BBA[b],
Stephen F. Brockmeier, MD[b],*

KEYWORDS

- Long head biceps tendon • Proximal biceps • Shoulder arthroscopy • SLAP repair
- Arthroscopic biceps tenodesis • Interference screw

KEY POINTS

- Arthroscopic proximal biceps reattachment (SLAP repair) is indicated for type II SLAP lesions in active younger patients with consistent history, physical examination, and imaging findings, and no identifiable concomitant pathologic abnormality.
- Outcomes after SLAP repair are largely favorable, although less successful outcomes have been demonstrated in certain populations, such as overhead athletes, patients older than 35 years of age, workers' compensation patients, and patients with concomitant shoulder pathologic abnormality.
- Biceps tenodesis is indicated for the management of proximal biceps pathologic abnormality, including SLAP tears and intrinsic biceps disorders, and may allow better ability to return to physical activity, improved cosmesis, and closer approximation of normal anatomy despite longer rehabilitation times and increased technical difficulty when compared with biceps tenotomy.
- Numerous arthroscopic fixation methods for biceps tenodesis have been described; however, the use of an interference screw or suture anchor construct is supported by most clinical evidence.
- Arthroscopic biceps tenodesis provides consistently favorable outcomes in terms of function and pain relief, without any long-term difference in clinical outcomes or complications when compared with open subpectoral tenodesis.

---

[a] Department of Sports Medicine and Shoulder Surgery, Hospital for Special Surgery, 535 East 70th Street, New York, NY 10021, USA; [b] Department of Orthopaedic Surgery, University of Virginia, 400 Ray C Hunt Drive, Suite 330, Charlottesville, VA 29903, USA
* Corresponding author.
E-mail address: sfb2e@virginia.edu

Clin Sports Med 35 (2016) 113–135
http://dx.doi.org/10.1016/j.csm.2015.08.001
0278-5919/16/$ – see front matter © 2016 Elsevier Inc. All rights reserved.

ARTHROSCOPIC SUPERIOR LABRUM ANTERIOR TO POSTERIOR REPAIR
Introduction

Arthroscopic proximal biceps reattachment (superior labrum anterior to posterior or SLAP repair) is a surgical technique used to address pathologic disruption of the anchor of the proximal long head of the biceps (LHB) tendon at its origin involving both the supraglenoid tubercle and the superior labrum.[1,2] First described by Andrews and colleagues[3] in 1985, disruption of the LHB anchor and superior labrum from the glenoid was termed a SLAP lesion by Snyder and colleagues[4] in 1990, who designated the first 4 anatomic classifications. Since that time, nearly 3 decades of research has established SLAP lesions as a source of shoulder pain. Currently, 10 different SLAP tear variants have been described as well as several implicated mechanisms of injury, including both traumatic injuries as well as repetitive overhead activity.[3,5–11] The proper management of SLAP lesions continues to evolve and remains controversial in certain populations stemming from the paucity of level I and II evidence, a multitude of identified confounding factors, and level III and IV studies with inconsistent and conflicting reported outcomes.

Indications/Contraindications

Although the accurate diagnosis of an SLAP lesion continues to be an area of debate, most would agree that a definitive diagnosis can be best made based on arthroscopic findings in the context of a combination of appropriate history, provocative tests, and imaging. Patient presentation can be variable, but common symptoms include pain localized to either the posterior or the anterior glenohumeral joint line. The pain is often provoked by certain activities or positions and is sometimes associated with mechanical catching in the joint and "dead-arm" episodes. In the overhead athlete population, pain can often be accompanied by fatigue, disordered shoulder mechanics, and diminished performance. Physical examination findings can be variable with several specialized tests that can be useful, including O'Brien's active compression test, the crank test, and biceps-specific tests such as the Speed's and Yergason's tests. No one examination finding has been shown to be acceptably specific for the diagnosis of an SLAP lesion. When SLAP pathologic abnormality is suspected based on history and examination, imaging in the form of an MRI with or without arthrography can further assist in the diagnosis. Before considering surgical repair, optimal management includes a trial of nonoperative treatment in those suspected of having an SLAP lesion.[8,12–14]

The evolving indications for arthroscopic repair of type II SLAP lesions depend on several patient factors, summarized in **Box 1**. In general, the patients with the strongest indications for and best expected outcomes after SLAP repair are active younger

---

Box 1
Indications for arthroscopic superior labrum anterior to posterior repair

- SLAP tears, typically type II
- Failure of conservative measures
- Significantly younger age (<35 years)
- Active athletic participation
- Absence of biceps tendon pathologic abnormality
- Overhead athletes

patients with consistent history, physical examination, and imaging findings, and no identifiable concomitant pathologic abnormality.[8,13,15]

Surgical Technique

Arthroscopic SLAP repair is most commonly carried out in the beach-chair position, although some surgeons prefer the lateral decubitus position. A standard diagnostic arthroscopy is completed using standard posterior and anterior portals. Once the diagnosis of an SLAP tear that is amenable to repair is confirmed, the surgeon can proceed with arthroscopic SLAP repair (**Fig. 1**).

- Portal placement
  - Portal placement is extremely important during SLAP repair to allow for an effective anatomic repair and limit additional iatrogenic trauma.
  - A high and somewhat lateral anterior portal is effective and allows a good angle for anchor placement. A cannula can further facilitate anchor placement through this portal.
  - Accessory portals are often necessary, which include a Neviaser portal (1 cm medial to the acromion in the triangle formed by the clavicle, acromion, and spine of the scapula) and the portal of Wilmington (1 cm lateral and anterior to the posterolateral corner of the acromion). It is both feasible and advisable to use a percutaneous technique through these 2 portal sites during SLAP repair to limit trauma to the surrounding soft tissue envelope (**Fig. 2A**).
- Preparation of SLAP tear site
  - To facilitate healing, an arthroscopic rasp is used to mobilize the lesion and free it from any scar or residual attachment.
  - A high-speed shaver or burr is then used to remove any cartilage or fibrinous material from the glenoid rim, to produce punctate-bleeding cortical bone, which will facilitate healing of the labrum.
- Anchor placement
  - The position and number of anchors for an arthroscopic SLAP repair can be variable and are determined based on the location and dimensions of the tear determined during diagnostic arthroscopy.

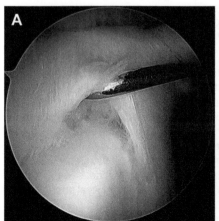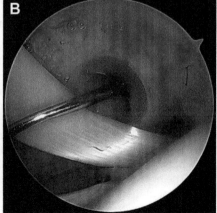

Fig. 1. Diagnostic arthroscopy of the right shoulder in the beach-chair position of a 26-year-old man with right shoulder pain demonstrates an SLAP tear (*A*) with normal-appearing biceps tendon (*B*).

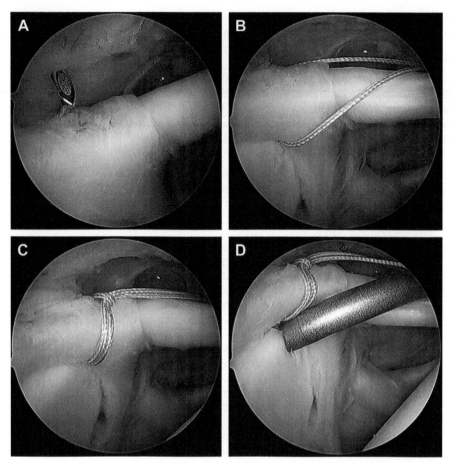

Fig. 2. The decision was made to proceed with SLAP tear given the normal appearance of the biceps tendon and patient's age. A spinal needle was placed through an accessory portal (*A*). A suture was passed through the labrum posterior to the biceps tendon after preparation of the tear (*B*). After the suture was tied (*C*), a position for the 2.4-mm knotless anchor was chosen posterior to the biceps tendon (*D*).

- For most SLAP lesions, the tear extends from the biceps anchor posteriorly, requiring 1 or 2 anchors placed posterior to the biceps anchor.
- The authors typically use small-diameter, biocomposite, absorbable, tap-in anchors because they are easier to control during insertion, limit the size of the perforation of the glenoid rim bone, and may diminish the risk of subsequent chondral injury due to anchor migration and prominence (see **Fig. 2**; **Fig. 3**).
- The authors further favor knotless anchor constructs in this region to limit the potential for abrasion or irritation related to knot prominence (see **Fig. 3**).
- The high and lateral anterior portal is used for the superior labral anchor placement at the 11:00/1:00 position.
- For posterior anchors, either a Wilmington or a posterolateral portal can be used similar to repair of a posterior labral tear.
- For most SLAP tears, posterior anchors alone are sufficient to stabilize the biceps-labral complex and normalize the peel-back phenomenon.

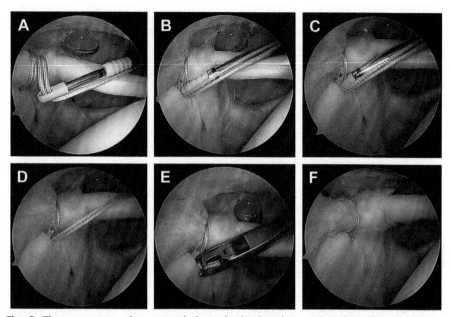

Fig. 3. The suture was then passed through the knotless anchor (*A*). The anchor was advanced into the previously drilled site (*B–D*). This was appropriately tensioned and then the free ends of the suture were cut (*E*). The superior labrum is reapproximated to its desired location (*F*).

- ○ If anterior anchors are required, extreme care must be taken to avoid incorporating the anterior capsule, middle glenohumeral ligament, or rotator interval structures.
- • Suture passage
  - ○ For each anchor that is placed, the medial suture (the suture closest to the labrum) is designated to be passed through the labrum.
  - ○ A suture-passing device with a wire loop or a spinal needle with a polydioxanone (PDS) suture is used to shuttle the suture through the labrum (see **Fig. 2**A–C).
  - ○ Sutures are then tied in a simple configuration with the postlimb of the suture superior to the labrum, to keep the knot away from the articular surface. Alternatively, both limbs of the suture can be passed, forming a horizontal mattress configuration, which is again tied superior to the labrum.
  - ○ Some surgeons prefer knotless techniques for SLAP repair. This technique involves passage of the suture (or a specialized broad tape suture) in either a simple or a horizontal fashion followed by preparation of the tract for the anchor, loading of the suture or tape into the knotless anchor, and finally tensioning and securing of the anchor to complete fixation (see **Figs. 2** and **3**).

Postoperative Care

The postoperative rehabilitation from arthroscopic SLAP repair used by the authors is divided into 4 distinct phases, which are summarized as:

- • Phase I: Protective phase (up to week 6)
  - ○ A sling is worn for 4 to 6 weeks
  - ○ Shoulder, elbow, and hand range of motion (ROM)

- Passive and gentle active-assisted ROM exercises
- By weeks 5 to 6, increase ROM and initiate limited active ROM
- Phase II: Moderate protection phase (weeks 7–12)
    - Can wean from sling
    - Begin isotonic rotator cuff strengthening with bands or weights
    - No biceps loading until week 10
    - May begin stretching exercises at 10 weeks if full ROM has not returned
- Phase III: Minimum protection phase (weeks 13–20)
    - Goals of this phase are nonpainful active and passive ROM, restoration of strength, power and endurance, and gradual initiation of functional activities
    - No throwing or overhead sport progression until week 16
    - Maintain full ROM
    - Increase intensity and decrease repetitions for most exercises
- Phase IV: Advanced strengthening phase (weeks 21–26)
    - Progress interval sports programs
    - Can begin throwing from a mound between weeks 24 and 28

Outcomes

The literature generally reports good to excellent outcomes in most patients undergoing arthroscopic proximal biceps reattachment (SLAP repair), although less successful outcomes have been demonstrated in certain populations, such as overhead athletes, patients older than 35 years of age, workers' compensation patients, and patients with concomitant shoulder pathologic abnormality. Outcome data of some of the recent literature are summarized in **Table 1**.[16–38] Recently, several authors have focused on the management of failed SLAP repairs manifesting as persistent postoperative pain or stiffness resistant to nonsurgical measures.[39–41] The literature suggests relatively poor revision outcomes and mostly supports the use of tenodesis for the management of SLAP repair failure.[42–45]

ARTHROSCOPIC PROXIMAL BICEPS TENODESIS
Introduction

LHB tenodesis has become an accepted and widely used surgical treatment option for patients with pain or disability attributed to a diseased or unstable biceps tendon who have failed conservative measures.[46–50] Numerous techniques for biceps tenodesis have been described, which can be generally classified into open[43,46,51–58] and arthroscopic[46,59–68] approaches. As tenodesis has increased in popularity, numerous fixation options have been described as well. However, regardless of technique, indication, or concomitant procedures, clinical outcomes after biceps tenodesis demonstrate generally favorable results, with excellent relief of pain, return to function, and return to work.[16,43–45,53,56,69–71]

Indications/Contraindications

Biceps tenodesis has emerged as a preferred technique for managing LHB pathologic abnormality in younger persons, athletes, laborers, and those wishing to avoid likely cosmetic deformity.[72] Indications for surgery include certain patients with SLAP tears, biceps tendinopathy, biceps subluxation or dislocation, partial biceps tendon tears, and in certain circumstances, biceps rupture that have failed appropriate conservative interventions. Considerations in the decision to perform biceps tenodesis as opposed to other procedures, such as biceps tenotomy, should include patient age, athletic participation, employment, and concern over cosmesis; however, the existing

Table 1
Superior labrum anterior to posterior repair clinical outcomes

Study	No. Patients	Mean Age	Mean Follow-Up	Population	Outcomes	Complications
General outcomes						
Boileau et al, 2009, AJSM, level III	25	37 y	2.9 y	Included 15 tenodesis and 10 repair patients with type II SLAP tears	Constant 83, increased from 65, 40% satisfaction; 20% return to sport/activities	4 (40%) revised to a tenodesis for repair failure
Brockmeier et al, 2009, JBJS, level IV	47	36 y	2.7 y	34 athletes, 13 nonathletes	ASES 97, from 62; L'Insalata 93, from 65 (P<.05), 87% good or excellent outcome; return to preinjury level of play 74% overall, 71% of overhead athletes, 92% in those reporting a discrete traumatic event vs 64% with atraumatic injury	4 refractory postop stiffness 2 reoperations
Oh et al, 2009, AJSM, level IV	60	43 y	2.7 y	—	93.3% UCLA good or excellent, pain visual analog scale 0.4, from 6; ASES 96, from 67.3; constant score 96.8, from 79.1; Return to sport 83%	None reported
Friel et al, 2010, JSES, level IV	48	33 y	3.4 y	27 athletes, 4 overhead laborers, 17 nonathletes	ASES 83, from 59. simple shoulder test 10.2 from 7.3; Improved ROM 79% G/E outcome (UCLA), RTP 62% overall, 59% of overhead athletes; no difference in subgroup analysis of overhead athletes, nonoverhead athletes, and nonathletes	4 reoperations: 2 revision repairs, 1 tenodesis, 1 tenotomy
Gorantla et al, 2010, Arthroscopy, systematic review	—	—	—	Systematic review of 12 studies from 1991 to 2009	Good and excellent results ranged from 40%–94% Return to sport ranged from 20%–94% for all athletes Return to sport averaged 64% for overhead athletes Mean UCLA 30.2–33.4, ASES 84–97, L'Insalata 85.1–93	—

(continued on next page)

Table 1
(continued)

Study	No. Patients	Mean Age	Mean Follow-Up	Population	Outcomes	Complications
Sayde et al, 2012, CORR, systematic review	—	—	—	Systematic review of 14 studies from 1991 to 2009	In 506 SLAP tears, 83% good to excellent satisfaction, 73% return to previous level of play In 198 overhead athletes, 63% return to play Higher satisfaction rates for anchor fixation (86%) vs tack fixation (74%) ($P<.003$)	—
Ek et al, 2014, JSES, level III	25	47 y	2.9 y	10 SLAP repair 15 Tenodesis (nonrandomized)	In repair group vs tenodesis group, no difference in ASES (93.5 vs 93.3, $P = .45$), satisfaction (90% vs 93%, $P = .45$), return to preinjury sport (60% vs 73%, $P = .66$), or pain VAS (0.8 vs 0.8, $P = .46$)	2 postop stiffness in repair group, 1 "Popeye" deformity in tenodesis group
Age-focused outcomes						
Neri et al, 2009, AJSM, level III	50	—	3 y	25 <40 y of age, 25 >40 y of age	Increase in ASES for both groups, no difference between groups (younger 91.4, from 59; older 87.1, from 54.6) Worse ASES with traumatic mechanism and osteoarthritis No difference in return to prior activity level (younger 80%, older 74%)	—
Alpert et al, 2010, AJSM, level III	52	—	2.3 y	21 <40 y of age, 31 >40 y of age	Younger group (n = 21) • 95% satisfied, 86% would have surgery again, shoulder 89% of normal Older group (n = 31) • 84% satisfied, 90% would have surgery again, shoulder 87% of normal No statistical difference in VAS, ASES, SST, SF-12	—

Study	N	Age	Follow-up	Details	Results	Complications
Denard et al, 2012, Arthroscopy, level IV	55	40 y	6.4 y	23 <40 y of age, 32 >40 y of age	Overall ASES 86.2 from 44.1, 87% good or excellent UCLA, 91% satisfaction, 82% return to normal sport or activity, G/E UCLA in 97% younger, 81% older, G/E UCLA in 65% workers' compensation, 95% non-workers' compensation	4 reoperations: 3 capsular releases, 1 unknown reoperation
Schroder et al, 2012, Arthroscopy, level IV	107	44 y	5.3 y	45 < 40 y of age, 62 > 40 y of age	Rowe score 92.1, from 62.8, 88% good or excellent satisfaction, 83.6% return to preinjury level of activity, 10/13 high level athletes RTP, Rowe score and satisfaction independent of age	13.1% had postop stiffness, 10.3% had reoperation
Provencher et al, 2013 AJSM, level III	179	32 y	3.4 y	Active military population	ASES 88, from 65; SANE 85, from 50. WOSI 82, from 54. 36.8% failure (defined as revision surgery, ASES <70, inability to return to sport or work). Age >36 y was only factor associated with increased incidence of failure. Mean age of failed group 39.2 y, healed group 29.7	28% reoperation (n = 42 tenodesis, 4 tenotomy, 4 debridement)
Denard et al, 2014, Orthopedics, level III	15	52 y	4.5 y	15 Tenodesis compared with 22 SLAP repair (avg age 45 y)	Repair group (n = 22) (mean age 45 y): • ASES 87.4, from 47.5; UCLA 31.2, from 18.5 • ROM recovery delay of 3 mo vs tenodesis group • 77% satisfaction and return to normal sport or activity vs 100% in tenodesis group (P = .067). Tenodesis group (n = 15) (mean age 52 y): • ASES 89.9, from 43.4; UCLA 32.7, from 19.0	2 refractory postop stiffness in repair group requiring capsular release
Erickson et al, 2014, AJSM, systematic review	—	—	—	Systematic review of 8 studies comparing younger (<40) and older (>40) patients	Mean ASES score 90.4 in patients <40 y, 84.6 in patients >40 y (P = .056). Mean UCLA score 32.4 in patients <40 y, 30.75 in patients >40 y (P = .667)	

(continued on next page)

Table 1
(continued)

Study	No. Patients	Mean Age	Mean Follow-Up	Population	Outcomes	Complications
Athlete-focused outcomes						
Neri et al, 2011, AJSM, level III	23	—	3.2 y	Elite overhead athletes	Return to preinjury level of play in 57%, return to play with pain limitation in 26%, no return to play in 17% Inability to return to preinjury level of play associated with concomitant partial thickness rotator cuff tear ($P = .006$)	—
Neuman et al, 2011, AJSM, level IV	30	24 y	3.5 y	Overhead athletes	ASES 87.9, KJOC 73.6 Subjectively returned to 84.1% of preinjury level with mean time to return to play of 11.7 mo 93.3% satisfied or very satisfied	—
Park et al, 2013, AJSM, level IV	24	23 y	3.8 y	Elite overhead athletes	ASES 87.1, from 55.8. VAS pain 2.0, from 5.7 Return to sport in 50% all overhead athletes, 38% in baseball player subgroup and 75% in other overhead athlete subgroup	—
Fedoriw et al, 2014, AJSM, level IV	68	24 y	—	Profession, baseball: 45 pitchers 23 position players	45 pitchers (mean age 23.7 y) • 18/45 with successful nonoperative therapy (40% RTP and 22% at previous level) • 27/45 failed nonoperative therapy and received surgery; 13/27 (48%) RTP and 7% at previous level 23 position players (mean age 23.9 y) • 9/23 with successful nonoperative therapy (39% RTP and 26% at previous level) • 13/23 failed nonoperative therapy and received surgery; 11/13 (85%) RTP and 54% at previous level	—

Concomitant rotator cuff pathologic abnormality outcomes

Study	N	Age	Follow-up	Groups	Outcomes	
Franceschi et al, 2008, AJSM, level I	31	62 y	5.2 y	31 RC repair + SLAP repair 32 RC repair + tenotomy (randomized)	RC repair + SLAP repair • UCLA 27.9, from 10.4 • 3/8 return to preinjury level of sport activities RC repair + tenotomy • UCLA 32.1, from 10.1 • 6/6 return to preinjury level of sport activities • Postop UCLA score, satisfaction, and ROM (FF, ER, IR) better than RC repair + SLAP repair (P<.05)	—
Abbot et al, 2009, AJSM, level II	24	53 y	2 y	24 RC repair + SLAP repair 24 RC repair + debridement (randomized)	RC repair + SLAP repair • UCLA 31, from 17.9. RC repair + debridement • UCLA 34, from 17.4. • Postop UCLA (total, pain, function) and 2 y ROM (ER, IR) better than RC repair + SLAP repair (P<.001)	—
Forsythe et al, 2010, 62 JBJS, level III	57 y	3.5 y		34 RC repair + SLAP repair 28 isolated RC repair	Concomitant SLAP repair + RC repair • ASES 96, from 23; normal constant 101, from 55.1 • 29/31 return to sports activities Isolated RC repair • ASES 92, from 34; normalized constant 96, from 61 • 16/18 return to sports activities	—

(continued on next page)

Table 1
(continued)

Study	No. Patients	Mean Age	Mean Follow-Up	Population	Outcomes	Complications
Kanatli et al, 2011, AOTS, level III	35	57 y	2.5 y	18 isolated SLAP repair 17 RC repair + SLAP repair	Isolated SLAP repair (mean age 58 y) • UCLA 31.2, from 11.5 • No significant difference in total UCLA score, but better function and satisfaction subscore vs RC repair + SLAP repair Concomitant RC repair + SLAP repair • UCLA 31, from 12.7	—
Kim et al, 2012, AJSM, level II	16	61 y	2 y	16 RC repair + SLAP repair 20 RC repair + tenotomy (large to massive RC tears)	RC repair + SLAP repair • SST 7.8, ASES 80.4, UCLA 26, FF ROM 133 RC repair + tenotomy • SST 9.3, ASES 88.6, UCLA 29.6, FF ROM 146 • All statistically significantly better than RCR + SLAP repair	—

Abbreviations: ASES, American Shoulder and Elbow Surgeon's Score; ER, external rotation; FF, forward flexion; IR, internal rotation; KJOC, Kerlan Jobe Orthopaedic Clinic score; RC, rotator cuff; RTP, return to play; SANE, Single Assessment Numeric Evaluation test; SF-12, Short Form – 12 Test; SST, simple shoulder test; UCLA, University of California Los Angeles Score; VAS, visual analog score; WOSI, Western Ontario Shoulder Instability Index.

evidence provides limited support in using these variables during the decision-making process (**Box 2**).[73] Although there is no consensus in the literature regarding tenotomy versus tenodesis, tenodesis allows better ability to return to physical activity, improved cosmesis, and closer approximation of normal anatomy despite longer rehabilitation times and increased technical difficulty.[12,47,51,53,59,62,74–78]

Surgical Technique

After the decision is made to proceed with biceps tenodesis based on a combination of patient factors, physical examination, and imaging findings, the patient is brought to the operating room. The patient may be positioned in either the lateral decubitus or the beach-chair position; the authors' preference is the beach-chair position for arthroscopic biceps tenodesis.

Three broad categories for arthroscopic biceps tenodesis have been described: high (at the entrance to or within the bicipital groove), low or suprapectoral (just above the pectoralis major tendon at the inferior extent of the bicipital groove), and soft tissue tenodesis, which is carried out most commonly high with suturing of the tendon remnant to the rotator interval tissue or incorporating it to the anterior extent of a concomitant rotator cuff repair.[58–66,68,79–86] The earliest descriptions of arthroscopic biceps tenodesis date to the early 2000s and recommended fixation just below the articular cartilage within the bicipital groove, leaving a large amount of residual biceps tendon proximal to the pectoralis major tendon.[59,64,65,80,87] More recently, largely over concern that retained tendon or tenosynovium can lead to persistent bicipital groove pain, some authors have advocated for a low suprapectoral position, just proximal to the pectoralis major tendon.[62,67]

The tendon can be fixed using a variety of methods, which include interference screws, suture anchors, or bicortical or unicortical button constructs. The authors currently favor an arthroscopic suprapectoral biceps tenodesis with an interference screw just proximal to the pectoralis major tendon insertion, which will be described later.

- Diagnostic arthroscopy and biceps tenotomy
    - A diagnostic arthroscopy is first performed using standard posterior and anterior arthroscopic portals (**Fig. 4**).
    - Once the decision is made to proceed with arthroscopic biceps tenodesis, the biceps tendon is tagged intra-articularly using a spinal needle or a PDS suture, to assist in maintenance of the length-tension relationship during the tenodesis procedure.
    - The tendon is then tenotomized from the superior labrum, and the biceps stump is debrided with an arthroscopic shaver.

Box 2
Indications for arthroscopic biceps tenodesis

- SLAP tears, biceps tendinosis/tendinopathy, biceps rupture
- Failure of conservative measures
- Younger age (compared with tenotomy)
- Athletic participation (compared with tenotomy)
- Patient worried about cosmesis
- Failed SLAP repair

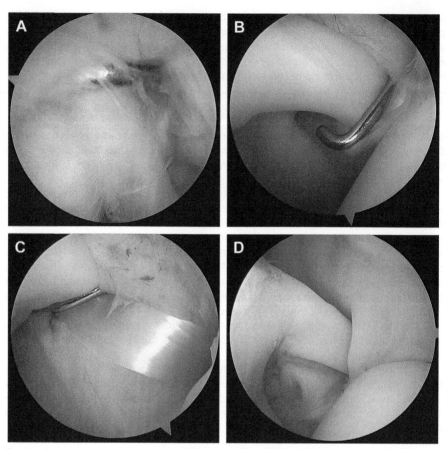

Fig. 4. Diagnostic arthroscopy of a right shoulder in a 56-year-old woman with right shoulder pain demonstrated an SLAP tear (*A*) with some mild long head biceps tendinosis (*B*). The remaining biceps tendon appeared intact (*C, D*).

- Arthroscopic suprapectoral tenodesis with an interference screw
  - For a suprapectoral tenodesis location, the arthroscopic instruments are then moved to the subacromial space and advanced into the more anterior and lateral subdeltoid space, which is developed deep to the deep deltoid fascia.
  - To facilitate access to the biceps tendon in the bicipital groove in the suprapectoral position, the arm is position in slight forward flexion, which can be maintained using one of many commercially available articulated limb positioners.
  - Moving anteriorly along the bicipital groove, the biceps tendon is identified just proximal to the pectoralis major insertion.
  - A suprapectoral location for the tenodesis site is identified just proximal to the pectoralis and cleared using electrocautery (**Fig. 5**A).
  - A motorized shaver is used to clear any remaining tenosynovium from the biceps tendon.
  - A guide pin for the tenodesis reamer is then inserted through a separate low anterior portal, which is localized using a spinal needle.

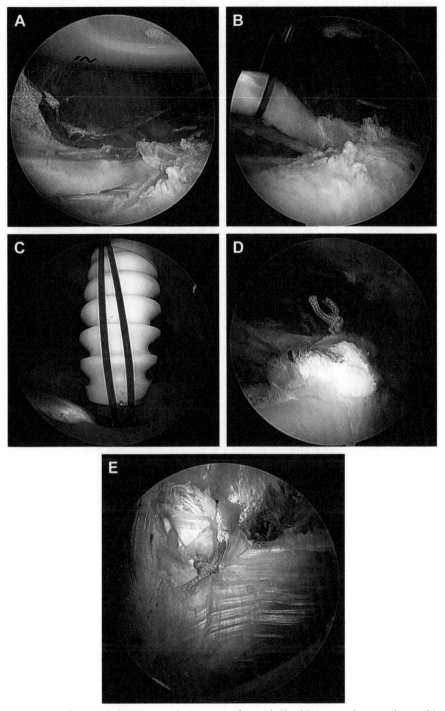

Fig. 5. An arthroscopic biceps tenodesis was performed. The biceps tendon was located in the bicipital groove just proximal to the pectoralis major tendon on the anterior humerus (*A*). A PDS suture was passed underneath the tendon to allow for control (*B*). After the tenodesis site was reamed, the tendon was then secured to the humerus using an interference screw (*C*, *D*). The final construct viewed from an anterior biceps portal demonstrates a tenodesis site just proximal to the insertion of the pectoralis major tendon (*E*).

Table 2
Arthroscopic tenodesis clinical outcomes

Study	No. Patients	Mean Age	Mean Follow-Up	Population	Technique	Outcomes	Complications
Boileau et al, 2002, Arthroscopy, level IV	43	63 y	1.4 y	3 patients with rotator cuff repair, 6 with isolated tenodesis, 34 with irreparable cuff tears	Interference screw	Improvement in constant score 43 points to 79 biceps strength 90% of contralateral side	2/43 patients with failure of tenodesis
Nord et al, 2005, Arthroscopy, level IV	11	60 y	2 y	Preliminary case series	Suture anchor	91% good/excellent results	1 patient with adhesive capsulitis
Boileau et al, 2009, level III	15	52 y	2.9 y	Included 15 tenodesis and 10 repair patients with type II SLAP tears	Interference screw	Constant score increased 30 points to 89; patient satisfaction 93%; 87% return to sport/activities	No failures in tenodesis group
Lutton et al, 2011, CORR, level IV	17	—	2.3 y	Isolated tenodesis procedures	Interference screw	Constant score improved 23 points to 81, ASES scores improved 29 points to 78	Persistent groove pain in 2 patients
Werner et al, 2014, Arthroscopy, level III	106	52 y	10 mo	Included 143 patients with open subpectoral tenodesis and 106 with arthroscopic	Interference screw for arthroscopic technique	No outcome scores reported; significantly increased rate of early postoperative stiffness in arthroscopic group (17.9%) compared with open subpectoral group (5.6%)	Increased postoperative stiffness in arthroscopic group

Study	N	Age	Follow-up	Description	Fixation technique	Outcomes	Complications
Werner et al, 2014, AJSM, level III	82	49 y	2.9 y	32 patients with arthroscopic tenodesis and 50 patients with open subpectoral tenodesis	Interference screw for both arthroscopic and open techniques	Final constant score: 91 final ASES: 90 final simple shoulder test: 10.4; no differences between scope and open groups	3/32 patients (9.4%) with postoperative stiffness in arthroscopic group
Scheibel et al, 2011, AJSM, level III	57	59 y	21 mo	Compared interference screw and soft tissue tenodesis; isolated LHB/SLAP pathologic abnormality	Interference screw (27 patients), soft tissue tenodesis (30 patients)	Average constant score 76.5; improved cosmesis with bony fixation compared with soft tissue tenodesis	Not reported
Gombera et al, 2015, AJSM, level III	46	57 y	30 mo	Compared 23 arthroscopic with 23 open subpectoral tenodesis	Interference screw for arthroscopic technique	No difference in ASES or patient satisfaction scores between groups	No complications for scope group; 2 complications in open group

Abbreviation: ASES, American Shoulder and Elbow Surgeon's Score.

○ The tenodesis site is then reamed, which is typically 0.5 mm greater than the size of the intended interference screw implant.

○ As the tendon and screw are inserted into the reamed site, the spinal needle or PDS suture, which secured the tendon intra-articularly, is released. Care is taken during tendon docking so as not to overtension the construct (see **Fig. 5B–E**).

○ For additional security, a suture can be sewn overtop to reinforce the fixation.

Complications and Management

Potential complications following arthroscopic biceps tenodesis are largely similar to those described for open subpectoral tenodesis and include persistent pain, fixation failure, infection, humerus fracture (if bone tunnels are drilled for interference screw fixation), and injuries to surrounding neurovascular structures, although the latter is likely much less common in arthroscopic tenodesis than in open procedures given the proximity of such structures.[55,88,89]

Specific to arthroscopic suprapectoral tenodesis, Werner and colleagues[90] noted an increased rate of early postoperative stiffness in patients who underwent the procedure (17.9%) compared with open subpectoral tenodesis (5.6%). This ROM discrepancy was not noted at minimum 2-year follow-up in a subsequent series published by the same investigators, indicating it to be an early phenomenon that responded well to physical therapy.[91]

Postoperative Care

The authors' postoperative rehabilitative protocol for an arthroscopic biceps tenodesis is identical to that described for an SLAP repair earlier in this article, using 4 phases of recovery.

Outcomes

Clinical outcomes of arthroscopic tenodesis methods are not as well-reported as those of open subpectoral tenodesis. Those authors publishing clinical results, though, have reported reasonable outcomes in terms of function and pain relief. The results of available studies with clinical or outcomes data after arthroscopic biceps tenodesis are reported in **Table 2**.[16,49,59,65,68,90–92]

SUMMARY

- Arthroscopic proximal biceps reattachment (SLAP repair) is indicated for type II SLAP lesions in active younger patients with consistent history, physical examination, and imaging findings, and no identifiable concomitant pathologic abnormality.
- SLAP repair is typically performed arthroscopically with the use of suture anchors and often through the use of accessory arthroscopic portals such as Neviaser or Wilmington.
- Outcomes after SLAP repair are largely favorable, although less successful outcomes have been demonstrated in certain populations such as overhead athletes, patients greater than 35 years of age, workers' compensation patients, and patients with concomitant shoulder pathologic abnormality.
- Biceps tenodesis is indicated for the management of proximal biceps pathologic abnormality, including SLAP tears and intrinsic biceps disorders, and may allow better ability to return to physical activity, improved cosmesis, and closer

approximation of normal anatomy despite longer rehabilitation times and increased technical difficulty when compared with biceps tenotomy.
- Numerous arthroscopic fixation methods for biceps tenodesis have been described; however, the use of an interference screw or suture anchor construct is supported by the most clinical evidence.
- Arthroscopic biceps tenodesis provides consistently favorable outcomes in terms of function and pain relief, without any long-term difference in clinical outcomes or complications when compared with open subpectoral tenodesis.

REFERENCES

1. Vangsness CT Jr, Jorgenson SS, Watson T, et al. The origin of the long head of the biceps from the scapula and glenoid labrum. An anatomical study of 100 shoulders. J Bone Joint Surg Br 1994;76:951–4.
2. Bain GI, Galley IJ, Singh C, et al. Anatomic study of the superior glenoid labrum. Clin Anat 2013;26:367–76.
3. Andrews JR, Carson WG Jr, McLeod WD. Glenoid labrum tears related to the long head of the biceps. Am J Sports Med 1985;13:337–41.
4. Snyder SJ, Karzel RP, Del Pizzo W, et al. SLAP lesions of the shoulder. Arthroscopy 1990;6:274–9.
5. Snyder SJ, Banas MP, Karzel RP. An analysis of 140 injuries to the superior glenoid labrum. J Shoulder Elbow Surg 1995;4:243–8.
6. Burkhart SS, Morgan CD, Kibler WB. The disabled throwing shoulder: spectrum of pathology. Part I: pathoanatomy and biomechanics. Arthroscopy 2003;19:404–20.
7. Burkhart SS, Morgan CD, Kibler WB. The disabled throwing shoulder: spectrum of pathology. Part II: evaluation and treatment of SLAP lesions in throwers. Arthroscopy 2003;19:531–9.
8. Keener JD, Brophy RH. Superior labral tears of the shoulder: pathogenesis, evaluation, and treatment. J Am Acad Orthop Surg 2009;17:627–37.
9. Maffet MW, Gartsman GM, Moseley B. Superior labrum-biceps tendon complex lesions of the shoulder. Am J Sports Med 1995;23:93–8.
10. Powell S, Nord K, Ryu R. The diagnosis, classification, and treatment of SLAP lesions. Oper Tech Sports Med 2004;12(2):99–110.
11. Morgan CD, Burkhart SS, Palmeri M, et al. Type II SLAP lesions: three subtypes and their relationships to superior instability and rotator cuff tears. Arthroscopy 1998;14:553–65.
12. Barber A, Field LD, Ryu R. Biceps tendon and superior labrum injuries: decision-making. J Bone Joint Surg Am 2007;89:1844–55.
13. McCormick F, Bhatia S, Chalmers P, et al. The management of type II superior labral anterior to posterior injuries. Orthop Clin North Am 2014;45:121–8.
14. Sando M, Henn RF, Guillermo A. Management of SLAP lesions: where are we in 2013?. In: Brockmeier S, Miller M, Guillermo A, editors. Surgery of shoulder instability. Berlin; Heidelberg: Springer; 2013. p. 125–40.
15. Burns JP, Bahk M, Snyder SJ. Superior labral tears: repair versus biceps tenodesis. J Shoulder Elbow Surg 2011;20:S2–8.
16. Boileau P, Parratte S, Chuinard C, et al. Arthroscopic treatment of isolated type II SLAP lesions: biceps tenodesis as an alternative to reinsertion. Am J Sports Med 2009;37:929–36.
17. Brockmeier SF, Voos JE, Williams RJ 3rd, et al. Outcomes after arthroscopic repair of type-II SLAP lesions. J Bone Joint Surg Am 2009;91:1595–603.

18. Oh JH, Lee HK, Kim JY, et al. Clinical and radiologic outcomes of arthroscopic glenoid labrum repair with the BioKnotless suture anchor. Am J Sports Med 2009;37:2340–8.

19. Friel NA, Karas V, Slabaugh MA, et al. Outcomes of type II superior labrum, anterior to posterior (SLAP) repair: prospective evaluation at a minimum two-year follow-up. J Shoulder Elbow Surg 2010;19:859–67.

20. Gorantla K, Gill C, Wright RW. The outcome of type II SLAP repair: a systematic review. Arthroscopy 2010;26:537–45.

21. Sayde WM, Cohen SB, Ciccotti MG, et al. Return to play after type II superior labral anterior-posterior lesion repairs in athletes: a systematic review. Clin Orthop Relat Res 2012;470:1595–600.

22. Ek ET, Shi LL, Tompson JD, et al. Surgical treatment of isolated type II superior labrum anterior-posterior (SLAP) lesions: repair versus biceps tenodesis. J Shoulder Elbow Surg 2014;23(7):1059–65.

23. Neri BR, Vollmer EA, Kvitne RS. Isolated type II superior labral anterior posterior lesions: age-related outcome of arthroscopic fixation. Am J Sports Med 2009;37: 937–42.

24. Alpert JM, Wuerz TH, O'Donnell TF, et al. The effect of age on the outcomes of arthroscopic repair of type II superior labral anterior and posterior lesions. Am J Sports Med 2010;38:2299–303.

25. Denard PJ, Ladermann A, Burkhart SS. Long-term outcome after arthroscopic repair of type II SLAP lesions: results according to age and workers' compensation status. Arthroscopy 2012;28:451–7.

26. Schroder CP, Skare O, Gjengedal E, et al. Long-term results after SLAP repair: a 5-year follow-up study of 107 patients with comparison of patients aged over and under 40 years. Arthroscopy 2012;28:1601–7.

27. Provencher MT, McCormick F, Dewing C, et al. A prospective analysis of 179 type 2 superior labrum anterior and posterior repairs: outcomes and factors associated with success and failure. Am J Sports Med 2013;41(4):880–6.

28. Denard PJ, Ladermann A, Parsley BK, et al. Arthroscopic biceps tenodesis compared with repair of isolated type II SLAP lesions in patients older than 35 years. Orthopedics 2014;37:e292–7.

29. Erickson J, Lavery K, Monica J, et al. Surgical treatment of symptomatic superior labrum anterior-posterior tears in patients older than 40 years: a systematic review. Am J Sports Med 2015;43(5):1274–82.

30. Neri BR, ElAttrache NS, Owsley KC, et al. Outcome of type II superior labral anterior posterior repairs in elite overhead athletes: effect of concomitant partial-thickness rotator cuff tears. Am J Sports Med 2011;39:114–20.

31. Neuman BJ, Boisvert CB, Reiter B, et al. Results of arthroscopic repair of type II superior labral anterior posterior lesions in overhead athletes: assessment of return to preinjury playing level and satisfaction. Am J Sports Med 2011;39:1883–8.

32. Park JY, Chung SW, Jeon SH, et al. Clinical and radiological outcomes of type 2 superior labral anterior posterior repairs in elite overhead athletes. Am J Sports Med 2013;41:1372–9.

33. Fedoriw WW, Ramkumar P, McCulloch PC, et al. Return to play after treatment of superior labral tears in professional baseball players. Am J Sports Med 2014;42: 1155–60.

34. Franceschi F, Longo UG, Ruzzini L, et al. No advantages in repairing a type II superior labrum anterior and posterior (SLAP) lesion when associated with rotator cuff repair in patients over age 50: a randomized controlled trial. Am J Sports Med 2008;36:247–53.

35. Abbot AE, Li X, Busconi BD. Arthroscopic treatment of concomitant superior labral anterior posterior (SLAP) lesions and rotator cuff tears in patients over the age of 45 years. Am J Sports Med 2009;37:1358–62.
36. Forsythe B, Guss D, Anthony SG, et al. Concomitant arthroscopic SLAP and rotator cuff repair. J Bone Joint Surg Am 2010;92:1362–9.
37. Kim SJ, Lee IS, Kim SH, et al. Arthroscopic repair of concomitant type II SLAP lesions in large to massive rotator cuff tears: comparison with biceps tenotomy. Am J Sports Med 2012;40:2786–93.
38. Kanatli U, Ozturk BY, Bolukbasi S. Arthroscopic repair of type II superior labrum anterior posterior (SLAP) lesions in patients over the age of 45 years: a prospective study. Arch Orthop Trauma Surg 2011;131:1107–13.
39. Werner BC, Brockmeier SF, Miller MD. Etiology, diagnosis, and management of failed SLAP repair. J Am Acad Orthop Surg 2014;22:554–65.
40. Weber SC. Surgical management of the failed SLAP repair. Sports Med Arthrosc 2010;18:162–6.
41. Katz LM, Hsu S, Miller SL, et al. Poor outcomes after SLAP repair: descriptive analysis and prognosis. Arthroscopy 2009;25:849–55.
42. Park S, Glousman RE. Outcomes of revision arthroscopic type II superior labral anterior posterior repairs. Am J Sports Med 2011;39:1290–4.
43. McCormick F, Nwachukwu BU, Solomon D, et al. The efficacy of biceps tenodesis in the treatment of failed superior labral anterior posterior repairs. Am J Sports Med 2014;42:820–5.
44. Werner BC, Pehlivan HC, Hart JM, et al. Biceps tenodesis is a viable option for salvage of failed SLAP repair. J Shoulder Elbow Surg 2014;23(8):e179–84.
45. Gupta AK, Bruce B, Klosterman EL, et al. Subpectoral biceps tenodesis for failed type II SLAP repair. Orthopedics 2013;36:e273–8.
46. Johannsen AM, Macalena JA, Carson EW, et al. Anatomic and radiographic comparison of arthroscopic suprapectoral and open subpectoral biceps tenodesis sites. Am J Sports Med 2013;41:2919–24.
47. Boileau P, Baque F, Valerio L, et al. Isolated arthroscopic biceps tenotomy or tenodesis improves symptoms in patients with massive irreparable rotator cuff tears. J Bone Joint Surg Am 2007;89:747–57.
48. Jarrett CD, McClelland WB Jr, Xerogeanes JW. Minimally invasive proximal biceps tenodesis: an anatomical study for optimal placement and safe surgical technique. J Shoulder Elbow Surg 2011;20:477–80.
49. Lutton DM, Gruson KI, Harrison AK, et al. Where to tenodese the biceps: proximal or distal? Clin Orthop Relat Res 2011;469:1050–5.
50. Mazzocca AD, McCarthy MB, Ledgard FA, et al. Histomorphologic changes of the long head of the biceps tendon in common shoulder pathologies. Arthroscopy 2013;29:972–81.
51. Mazzocca AD, Bicos J, Santangelo S, et al. The biomechanical evaluation of four fixation techniques for proximal biceps tenodesis. Arthroscopy 2005;21:1296–306.
52. Mazzocca AD, Rios CG, Romeo AA, et al. Subpectoral biceps tenodesis with interference screw fixation. Arthroscopy 2005;21:896.
53. Mazzocca AD, Cote MP, Arciero CL, et al. Clinical outcomes after subpectoral biceps tenodesis with an interference screw. Am J Sports Med 2008;36:1922–9.
54. Millett PJ, Sanders B, Gobezie R, et al. Interference screw vs. suture anchor fixation for open subpectoral biceps tenodesis: does it matter? BMC Musculoskelet Disord 2008;9:121.

55. Provencher MT, LeClere LE, Romeo AA. Subpectoral biceps tenodesis. Sports Med Arthrosc 2008;16:170–6.
56. Nho SJ, Frank RM, Reiff SN, et al. Arthroscopic repair of anterosuperior rotator cuff tears combined with open biceps tenodesis. Arthroscopy 2010;26:1667–74.
57. Dickens JF, Kilcoyne KG, Tintle SM, et al. Subpectoral biceps tenodesis: an anatomic study and evaluation of at-risk structures. Am J Sports Med 2012;40: 2337–41.
58. Patzer T, Santo G, Olender GD, et al. Suprapectoral or subpectoral position for biceps tenodesis: biomechanical comparison of four different techniques in both positions. J Shoulder Elbow Surg 2012;21:116–25.
59. Boileau P, Krishnan SG, Coste JS, et al. Arthroscopic biceps tenodesis: a new technique using bioabsorbable interference screw fixation. Arthroscopy 2002; 18:1002–12.
60. Ahmad CS, ElAttrache NS. Arthroscopic biceps tenodesis. Orthop Clin North Am 2003;34:499–506.
61. Sekiya JK, Elkousy HA, Rodosky MW. Arthroscopic biceps tenodesis using the percutaneous intra-articular transtendon technique. Arthroscopy 2003;19:1137–41.
62. Romeo AA, Mazzocca AD, Tauro JC. Arthroscopic biceps tenodesis. Arthroscopy 2004;20:206–13.
63. Boileau P, Neyton L. Arthroscopic tenodesis for lesions of the long head of the biceps. Oper Orthop Traumatol 2005;17:601–23.
64. Kim SH, Yoo JC. Arthroscopic biceps tenodesis using interference screw: end-tunnel technique. Arthroscopy 2005;21:1405.
65. Nord KD, Smith GB, Mauck BM. Arthroscopic biceps tenodesis using suture anchors through the subclavian portal. Arthroscopy 2005;21:248–52.
66. Verma NN, Drakos M, O'Brien SJ. Arthroscopic transfer of the long head biceps to the conjoint tendon. Arthroscopy 2005;21:764.
67. David TS, Schildhorn JC. Arthroscopic suprapectoral tenodesis of the long head biceps: reproducing an anatomic length-tension relationship. Arthrosc Tech 2012;1:e127–32.
68. Scheibel M, Schroder RJ, Chen J, et al. Arthroscopic soft tissue tenodesis versus bony fixation anchor tenodesis of the long head of the biceps tendon. Am J Sports Med 2011;39:1046–52.
69. Lee HI, Shon MS, Koh KH, et al. Clinical and radiologic results of arthroscopic biceps tenodesis with suture anchor in the setting of rotator cuff tear. J Shoulder Elbow Surg 2014;23:e53–60.
70. Skare O, Schroder CP, Reikeras O, et al. Efficacy of labral repair, biceps tenodesis, and diagnostic arthroscopy for SLAP lesions of the shoulder: a randomised controlled trial. BMC Musculoskelet Disord 2010;11:228.
71. Sanders B, Lavery KP, Pennington S, et al. Clinical success of biceps tenodesis with and without release of the transverse humeral ligament. J Shoulder Elbow Surg 2012;21:66–71.
72. Nho SJ, Strauss EJ, Lenart BA, et al. Long head of the biceps tendinopathy: diagnosis and management. J Am Acad Orthop Surg 2010;18:645–56.
73. Slenker NR, Lawson K, Ciccotti MG, et al. Biceps tenotomy versus tenodesis: clinical outcomes. Arthroscopy 2012;28:576–82.
74. Hsu AR, Ghodadra NS, Provencher MT, et al. Biceps tenotomy versus tenodesis: a review of clinical outcomes and biomechanical results. J Shoulder Elbow Surg 2011;20:326–32.
75. Osbahr DC, Diamond AB, Speer KP. The cosmetic appearance of the biceps muscle after long-head tenotomy versus tenodesis. Arthroscopy 2002;18:483–7.

76. Wittstein JR, Queen R, Abbey A, et al. Isokinetic strength, endurance, and subjective outcomes after biceps tenotomy versus tenodesis: a postoperative study. Am J Sports Med 2011;39:857–65.
77. Koh KH, Ahn JH, Kim SM, et al. Treatment of biceps tendon lesions in the setting of rotator cuff tears: prospective cohort study of tenotomy versus tenodesis. Am J Sports Med 2010;38:1584–90.
78. Wolf RS, Zheng N, Weichel D. Long head biceps tenotomy versus tenodesis: a cadaveric biomechanical analysis. Arthroscopy 2005;21:182–5.
79. Klepps S, Hazrati Y, Flatow E. Arthroscopic biceps tenodesis. Arthroscopy 2002; 18:1040–5.
80. Lo IK, Burkhart SS. Arthroscopic biceps tenodesis using a bioabsorbable interference screw. Arthroscopy 2004;20:85–95.
81. Elkousy HA, Fluhme DJ, O'Connor DP, et al. Arthroscopic biceps tenodesis using the percutaneous, intra-articular trans-tendon technique: preliminary results. Orthopedics 2005;28:1316–9.
82. Castagna A, Conti M, Mouhsine E, et al. Arthroscopic biceps tendon tenodesis: the anchorage technical note. Knee Surg Sports Traumatol Arthrosc 2006;14: 581–5.
83. Hapa O, Gunay C, Komurcu E, et al. Biceps tenodesis with interference screw: cyclic testing of different techniques. Knee Surg Sports Traumatol Arthrosc 2010;18:1779–84.
84. Patzer T, Rundic JM, Bobrowitsch E, et al. Biomechanical comparison of arthroscopically performable techniques for suprapectoral biceps tenodesis. Arthroscopy 2011;27:1036–47.
85. Franceschi F, Longo UG, Ruzzini L, et al. Soft tissue tenodesis of the long head of the biceps tendon associated to the roman bridge repair. BMC Musculoskelet Disord 2008;9:78.
86. Lafosse L, Shah AA, Butler RB, et al. Arthroscopic biceps tenodesis to supraspinatus tendon: technical note. Am J Orthop (Belle Mead NJ) 2011;40:345–7.
87. Gartsman GM, Hammerman SM. Arthroscopic biceps tenodesis. Operative technique. Arthroscopy 2000;16:550–2.
88. Nho SJ, Reiff SN, Verma NN, et al. Complications associated with subpectoral biceps tenodesis: low rates of incidence following surgery. J Shoulder Elbow Surg 2010;19:764–8.
89. Rhee PC, Spinner RJ, Bishop AT, et al. Iatrogenic brachial plexus injuries associated with open subpectoral biceps tenodesis: a report of 4 cases. Am J Sports Med 2013;41:2048–53.
90. Werner BC, Pehlivan HC, Hart JM, et al. Increased incidence of postoperative stiffness after arthroscopic compared with open biceps tenodesis. Arthroscopy 2014;30(9):1075–84.
91. Werner BC, Evans CL, Holzgrefe RE, et al. Arthroscopic suprapectoral and open subpectoral biceps tenodesis: a comparison of minimum 2-year clinical outcomes. Am J Sports Med 2014;42:2583–90.
92. Gombera MM, Kahlenberg CA, Nair R, et al. All-arthroscopic suprapectoral versus open subpectoral tenodesis of the long head of the biceps brachii. Am J Sports Med 2015;43:1077–83.

Open Subpectoral Tenodesis of the Proximal Biceps

Andreas Voss, MD[a], Simone Cerciello, MD[b], Justin Yang, MD[a],
Knut Beitzel, MA, MD[c], Mark P. Cote, PT, DPT, MSCTR[a],
Augustus D. Mazzocca, MS, MD[d],*

KEYWORDS

- Subpectoral • Proximal biceps • Tenodesis • Open • Long head of the biceps

KEY POINTS

- A safe and reproducible blunt dissection of the pectoralis major tendon allows access to the biceps directly inferior.
- It is important to have a sufficient lateral retraction of the pectoralis major muscle-tendon-unit and medial retraction of the conjoined tendons to permit access to the bicipital groove.
- Create an 8 mm bone tunnel by an 8-mm canulated reamer in the center portion of the proximal humerus to prevent fractures.
- The visual examination and palpation of the tenodesis are a major key point to confirm the screw is flush with the cortex and the tendon is in correct position.

INTRODUCTION

In many cases, the intra-articular portion of the long head of the biceps tendon (LHBT) is the origin of shoulder pain due to instability within the bicipital groove, tendinosis, or a superior labral tear from anterior to posterior (SLAP) lesion at its origin. At the

Funding source: None (A. Voss, J. Yang, S. Cerciello, K. Beitzel, M.P. Cote). Arhtrex Inc, Naples, FL, USA (Consultant and Research) (A.D. Mazzocca).
Conflict of Interest: None (A. Voss, J. Yang, S. Cerciello, K. Beitzel, M.P. Cote). The University of Connecticut Health Center/UConn Musculoskeletal Institute has received research funding from Arthrex (Naples, FL). The company had no influence on study design, data collection, or interpretation of the results or on the final article (A.D. Mazzocca).
[a] Department of Orthopaedic Surgery, UConn Musculoskeletal Institute, University of Connecticut, 263 Farmington Avenue, Farmington, CT 06034, USA; [b] Department of Geriatrics, Neurosciences and Orthopaedics, Policlinico Agostino Gemelli, Catholic University of Rome, Largo Francesco Vito 1, Rome 00135, Italy; [c] Department of Orthopaedic Sports Medicine, Technical University Munich, Ismaninger Street 22, Munich 81675, Germany; [d] Department of Orthopaedic Surgery, UConn Musculoskeletal Institute, UConn Health, University of Connecticut, 263 Farmington Avenue, Farmington, CT 06034, USA
* Corresponding author.
E-mail address: mazzocca@uchc.edu

beginning of nineteenth century, Gilcreest[1] first described a tenodesis as a treatment to address these pathologies. In the 1980s, we observed that some patients with severe shoulder pain and rotator cuff tear often experienced relief of pain after a spontaneous rupture of the biceps tendon. Following this clinical observation, we started to perform a release of the biceps tendon under arthroscopic control in patients with a pathologically altered tendon associated with massive, nonreparable cuff tears to improve their symptoms.[2]

The LHBT has also been evaluated histologically. In common shoulder pathologies, the LHBT has demonstrated a greater degree of degeneration of the intra-articular tendon compared with the extra-articular portion.[3] In patients with LHBT instability, tendinosis, or degenerative joint disease, the proximal or intra-articular LHBT demonstrates significantly poorer organization as well as increased proteoglycan content compared with normal LHBTs. In contrast, the distal or extra-articular portion of the tendon has a greater degree of collagen organization with less proteoglycan content, suggesting a healthy tendon.[3] Theses findings indicate a greater degree of degeneration in the proximal part of the tendon, lending support for subpectoral biceps tenodesis.

A potential advantage of the open subpectoral biceps tenodesis compared with the arthroscopic suprapectoral technique is avoiding additional risk of impingement due to the proximal biceps stump created at the bicipital groove. Furthermore, Alpantaki and colleagues[4] demonstrated the presence of a large network of sensory nerve fibers in the biceps tendon, with greater sensory innervation present in the more proximal aspect of the tendon. Given these findings, the goal of the open subpectoral tenodesis is to remove the proximal biceps tendon to reduce the pain stimuli and preserve the physiologic shape of the upper arm.

INDICATIONS/CONTRAINDICATIONS

Conservative treatment should be considered primarily when pathology of the LHBT is diagnosed, except for biceps tendon instability or in the presence of a concomitant repairable rotator cuff tear.[5] For patients who fail conservative treatment, operative intervention is indicated. Compared with simple tenotomy, a biceps tenodesis offers a more favorable cosmetic result by maintaining the physiologic shape of the upper arm.[6] **Table 1** illustrates the indications and contraindications for open subpectoral biceps tenodesis.[5–11]

SURGICAL TECHNIQUES

Several techniques for subpectoral biceps tenodesis have been described. They all include preliminary arthroscopic evaluation of the glenohumeral joint to assess the integrity of the biceps anchor, the biceps pulley, and the tendon itself. An initial arthroscopic tenotomy is performed, regardless of technique.

Bone Tunnel Technique

The bone tunnel technique was initially described by Snyder[12] and subsequently popularized by several investigators. Said and colleagues[13] described their technique in a series of 30 patients. The procedure starts with a longitudinal incision starting 1 cm proximal to the inferior border of the pectoralis tendon and extending distally for 3 cm along the medial aspect of the arm. The tendon of the biceps is identified through blunt dissection. Approximately 20 mm to 25 mm of tendon (from the musculotendinous junction [MTJ]) is left in place to ensure the correct tendon length and weaved with Vicryl no. 2 suture (Ethicon, West Somerville, NJ, USA) using a

Table 1 Indications and contraindications for open subpectoral tenodesis of the long head of the biceps tendon	
Indications	**Contraindication**
• Chronic atrophic changes in the LHBT	• Severe osteoporotic bone
• Painful and therapy-resistant tenosynovitis	• Implants in the area of the tenodesis
• Symptomatic intra-articular partial tears (>25%–50%) of the LHBT	(humeral nail or humeral stem)
• Additional treatment during rotator cuff repair, especially during repair of the subscapularis tendon to protect the construct	• Tumors or cysts in the area of the bicipital groove and the proximal humeral shaft • Patient cosmetic concerns
• Biceps instability	
• SLAP lesions in elderly patients	
• Painful and hyperthrophic LHBT with secondary impingement and asymmetrical loss of elevation (hourglass biceps)	
• Subpectoral biceps pain	

whipstitch technique. Two 4.5-mm holes are drilled in the anterior humeral cortex with the distal hole at the level of the lower border of the pectoralis major and the superior hole 1.5 cm to 2 cm proximally. The tendon is pulled from the distal hole through the proximal hole, tensioned, looped distally, and then sutured into the muscle itself. At a follow-up ranging from 12 to 18 months, average Constant and Oxford shoulder scores improved from 39.03 and 21.3, respectively, to 76.43 and 44.8, respectively.

Kane and colleagues[14] described a similar technique in a series of 102 patients. The technique uses a 7.5-mm unicortical tunnel drilled just superior to the inferior margin of the pectoralis tendon; 2 additional 2.4-mm tunnels are prepared distal to the first hole. Two shuttle sutures are passed from the small holes to the central hole. The biceps tendon is prepared in a standard fashion, removing the excess tendon, leaving 1 cm to 2 cm of tendon from the MTJ, and placing a locking Krackow stitch at the junction. The 2 free ends are passed into the central hole and retrieved from the distal holes. The sutures are then pulled to dock the tendon in the central hole within the intramedullary canal and tied. In their series, 98% of patients were satisfied with the operation.

Cortical Button Technique

Snir and colleagues[15] described a similar technique and used a cortical button to provide tendon fixation. The biceps and location for the tenodesis are identified through a standard subpectoral approach. The tendon is prepared with whipstitches beginning at the MTJ and extending 1.5 cm proximally. The location of the bone tunnel is identified at the most distal aspect of the bicipital groove. A 3.2-mm Kirschner (K)-wire is then placed through the anterior cortex. A unicortical hole is drilled over the K-wire, choosing a slightly larger diameter than the tendon itself (ie, 5-mm drill for a 4.5-mm tendon). The posterior cortex is then drilled with the 3.2-mm K-wire to allow for the passage of the cortical button. The cortical button is loaded onto the BicepsButton (Arthrex, Naples, Florida) deployment device and passed deep to the posterior cortex of the humerus. The device is removed as soon as the button clears the posterior cortex. The tendon is then shuttled into the tunnel by pulling the sutures until it reaches the posterior cortex. The free end of 1 suture is passed through the tendon and tied to the second to augment the strength of the construct.

Keyhole Technique

The keyhole technique for biceps tenodesis was initially described by Froimson and O.[16] According to the investigators, the proximal end of the biceps tendon was rolled into a ball and was sutured with no. 2 Ethibond (Ethicon, West Somerville, NJ, USA) to achieve a solid mass. A keyhole was prepared into the bicipital groove with a small burr. The tendon was inserted into the keyhole and pulled distally to lock the tendon mass. Although the original technique was performed through an open approach at the distal aspect of the groove, some reports demonstrate the possibility of humerus fracture with utilization of this technique,[17] and this has led some surgeons to prefer a more proximal tenodesis.[18,19]

Suture Anchor Technique

Suture anchor fixation requires small holes (2–3 mm), but the drawback to this technique is that the tendon must heal to the surface of the humeral cortex instead of within the canal. Sanders and colleagues[20] described his technique of fixation with a single double-loaded suture anchor. After the anterior aspect of the humeral cortex is prepared at the proposed location, the anchor is positioned at the inferior border of the pectoralis major insertion. The tendon is fixed with 2 locking lasso-loop stitches and secured to the anterior humeral cortex. A similar technique was described by Scully and colleagues.[21] Through a mini-open approach, the location for the anchor is identified approximately 1 cm proximal to the distal aspect of the pectoralis major insertion. The socket for the double-loaded anchor is prepared with a 2.9-mm drill. The tendon is prepared with 3 to 4 locked Krackow stitches beginning 1 cm proximal to the MTJ. The free ends of both sutures are used to shuttle the tendon down to the anchor and are tied, securing the tendon to the anterior humeral cortex.

Su and colleagues[22] recently described his technique of suture anchor fixation. At the desired location 2 cm proximal to the inferior border of the pectoralis major insertion, the periosteum is reflected. A hole in the anterior cortex is prepared with a 5-mm drill. The posterior humeral cortex is drilled with a 1.3-mm drill. The suture anchor is then positioned just beyond the posterior cortex and blocked by pulling the 2 suture limbs. One end is used to perform a modified rolling hitch suture around the tendon, and the other end is used to shuttle the tendon into the anterior cortical hole by gently pulling it until it reaches the posterior humeral cortex. The sutured limb is passed again through the tendon (at the exit of the tunnel) to reinforce the fixation.

Interference Screw Technique

Mazzocca and colleagues[23] popularized fixation with interference screws. This option allows intramedullary healing of the tendon and used a combination of the techniques described previously.

PREPARATION AND PATIENT POSITIONING

Prior to surgery patients receive an antiseptic and antimicrobial skin cleanser (chlorhexidine gluconate solution). Patients are instructed to wash the involved shoulder with the cleanser 2 days before, the day before, and the morning of surgery in an effort to reduce the risk of infection. After induction of anesthesia, the patient is placed into a beach chair position and the surgical site is washed with chlorhexidine gluconate and isopropyl alcohol and 2 g of cefazolin is given intravenously for infection prophylaxis.

The arm is fixed with a Trimano specialized arm-holder (Arthrex). The arm is positioned in 30° to 45° of forward flexion, abducted 20° to 30°, and slightly externally rotated (**Figs. 1** and **2**).

Prior to incision the anatomic landmarks (the acromion, the clavicle, the acromioclavicular joint, and the coracoid) are marked along with the proposed portal sites. For both the diagnostic arthroscopy and the LHBT release, a standard posterior portal with an anterior-superior working portal is preferable (**Fig. 3**).

For the open biceps tenodesis, the skin incision is marked longitudinally in the patient's axillary fold over the pectoralis major insertion (**Fig. 4**).

SURGICAL APPROACH

There are various anatomic landmarks to be considered during this procedure. LaFrance and colleagues[24] reported in a cadaveric study about the MTJ of the biceps, which can begin more proximal than assumed. Furthermore, they demonstrated anatomic variations of the biceps. They recommend a tenodesis by placing the MTJ approximately 3 cm distal to the inferior border of the pectoralis major insertion. The position of the tenodesis relative to the MTJ is important because it dictates the tension on the LHBT, which can affect cosmesis.[24]

Sethi and colleagues[25] summarized and evaluated the risk of neurologic injury in a cadaveric study with a bicortical method using the same anatomic landmarks as described by Mazzocca and colleagues,[23] with a tenodesis insertion 1 cm proximal to the distal border of the pectoralis major tendon (**Table 2**), and found it a safe procedure. Dickens and colleagues[26] also investigated the adjacent neurovascular structures using the same surgical approach as described previously, but retractors were positioned on the medial and lateral borders of the humerus to expose the insertion point for the tenodesis. **Table 2** illustrates the different results found by the 2 investigators. Dickens and colleagues[26] measured the proximity of the neurovascular structures in different arm positions including internal and external rotation of the humerus (±45°) and concluded that there is a greater risk of injury to these structures during subpectoral biceps tenodesis with internal rotation and with the use of a medial retractor. These differences may be explained by a variation of specimen size used in these 2 studies and the variability of the pectoralis major footprint as shown in a

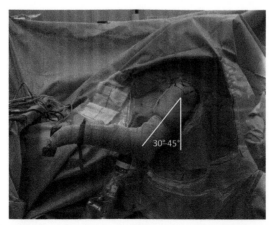

Fig. 1. Beach chair position with a forward elevated arm to 30° to 45° in reference to an upright position.

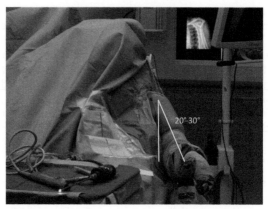

Fig. 2. The arm is slightly abducted 20° to 30° and externally rotated to access the field of interest and to place the pectoralis major tendon under tension.

cadaveric study by Carey and Owens,[27] which showed a mean proximal to distal length of 72.3 mm ± 12.3 mm and a range of 50.8 mm to 87.4 mm.

After a diagnostic arthroscopy and the documentation of additional glenohumeral pathology, the LHBT is tenotomized close to the base at the superior rim of the glenoid with a meniscal biter, an arthroscopic scissor, or a radiofrequency ablation device (**Fig. 5**). This procedure can be followed by additional arthroscopic treatments if required.

After the glenohumeral joint management has been complete, attention is turned toward the upper arm. The skin incision is made and blunt dissection is carried out using the surgeon's finger to explore the interval between the pectoralis major muscle tendon and the proximal aspect of the short head of the biceps muscle belly (**Fig. 6**). It is important to feel the LHBT within the bicipital groove. The pectoralis major tendon is retracted superiorly and laterally, and the short head of the biceps is carefully retracted medially. This exposes the bicipital groove, allowing the surgeon to pull the LHBT into the wound.

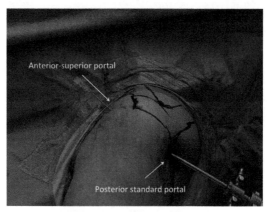

Fig. 3. To access the glenohumeral joint, a standard posterior portal is used for visualization and an anterior-superior portal for instrumentation.

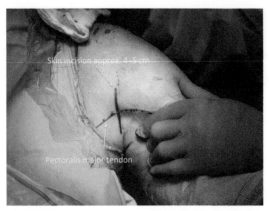

Fig. 4. By externally rotating the arm, the pectoralis major tendon comes under tension (*blue horizontal line*) and allows access to the axillary fold for the skin incision (*violet vertical line*).

A guide pin is placed within the center of the bicipital groove with the pin perpendicular to the humeral cortex (**Fig. 7**). It is important to elevate the pectoralis major tendon enough to permit sufficient access to the bicipital groove to expose the tenodesis site (**Fig. 8**). Subsequently, an 8-mm unicortical hole is drilled using an 8-mm cannulated reamer to prepare the cortex (**Fig. 9**). After reaming, the surgical field is irrigated to remove bone debris.

The LHBT is stitched (whipstitch or Krackow suture configuration) starting 2 cm from the MTJ. The excess tendon is cut and a knot is tied with the 2 suture ends (**Fig. 10**). One of the sutures is loaded through the biceps tenodesis driver (Arthrex), and the other end is left free (**Fig. 11**). An 8 × 12 mm polyetheretherketone screw (Arthrex) is then deployed along with the tendon into the previously drilled 8-mm hole until the screw is flush with the humeral cortex (**Figs. 12** and **13**). The 2 ends of the suture are tied over the screw, providing additional fixation to the construct.

Table 2
Differences regarding proximity of subpectoral biceps tenodesis to neurovascular structures

Neurovascular Structure	Sethi et al,[25] 2015			Dickens et al,[26] 2012		
	Position	Mean ± SD (mm)	Range (mm)	Position	Mean ± SD (mm)	Range (mm)
Radial nerve	*	48.0 ± 10.7	31.7–60.8	N	16.6 ± 5.9	10–32
Axillary nerve	*	36.7 ± 11.2	20.5–63.5	N	33.8 ± 6.9	20–45
Musculocutaneous nerve	*	37.4 ± 11.2	14.0–43.1	N	10.1 ± 3.3	6–18
				I	8.1 ± 3.3	3–16
				E	19.4 ± 8.2	11–32
Median nerve	*	—	—	N	27.6 ± 5.5	18–49
Deep brachial artery	*	—	—	N	14.5 ± 6.0	9–30
Brachial vein	*	—	—	N	32.5 ± 6.4	19–45
Brachial artery	*	—	—	N	32 ± 5.7	20–43

Abbreviations: *, not mentioned; E, external rotation; I, internal rotation; N, neutral.

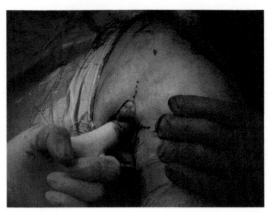

Fig. 5. The skin incision is followed by a safe and reproducible blunt dissection of the pectoralis major tendon until the bicipital groove and the LHBT are exposed.

Fig. 14 shows an arthroscopic view of the flush tenodesis screw and the insertion of the LHBT.

The open subpectoral biceps tenodesis site is irrigated and 1 g of vancomycin powder is placed into the wound for prophylaxis against *Propionibacterium acnes* prior to wound closure. The wound is closed using a 3 to 0 Monocryl (Ethicon, West Somerville, NJ, USA) in interrupted subcuticular fashion, followed by a topical skin closure adhesive, Dermabond (Ethicon, Norwood, Massachusetts). The wound is covered by Steri-Strips (3M, St. Paul, Minnesota), and the patient is placed into a sling prior to waking.

BIOMECHANICS

The literature suggests that subpectoral biceps tenodesis with interference screw fixation offers superior biomechanical strength compared with other techniques. In a study of 42 cadaveric specimens comparing suture anchors and interference screws, an axial cyclic load with 100 cycles, 1-Hz frequency, and 50-N maximal load was

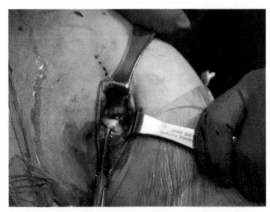

Fig. 6. By retracting the lateral part of the wound and the pectoralis major tendon, the LHBT can be pulled out by using a right-angled clamp. This is done before placing a blunt hohmann retractor, because the biceps might be incarcerated and not in the field.

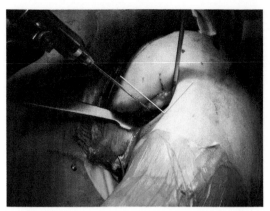

Fig. 7. A guide pin is used to drill a unicortical hole in the ventral aspect of the cortex within the bicipital groove. The pin is placed perpendicular to the humerus (*yellow lines*) and directly in the center of the groove. Care must be taken to avoid being too lateral or medial, which can weaken the cortex and predispose to postoperative humerus fracture.

applied; the interference screw had significantly higher ultimate failure load.[28] In another cadaveric study comparing suture anchors and interference screw fixation, the interference screw was significantly stronger than the suture anchor construct[29]; the ultimate failure load with dual anchors was similar to interference screw fixation. In another cadaveric study, interference screw fixation had better pullout strength than the dual anchor technique.[30] The suture anchors in this study all failed at a mean 135 N, compared with interference screw failure at 233 N. The senior author's study compared 4 fixation methods in a human cadaver model including subpectoral interference screw, bone tunnel suture fixation, arthroscopic suprapectoral tenodesis with interference screw fixation, and arthroscopic tenodesis with suture anchor fixation. After 5000 cycles with a 100-N load cycled at 1 Hz, only subpectoral biceps tenodesis with bone tunnel suture fixation showed statistically significant displacement compared with other fixation methods, suggesting that it is less stable with cyclic loading. There was no statistically significant difference in the mean ultimate failure

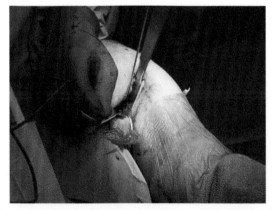

Fig. 8. The most important step in this procedure is the sufficiently elevating the pectoralis major tendon to permit access to the bicipital groove.

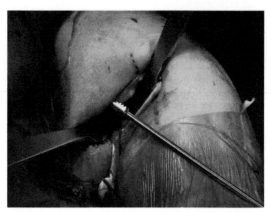

Fig. 9. After unicortical drilling, an 8-mm tap is used to prepare the proximal cortex for screw placement.

loads among the groups. These results show that the subpectoral interference screw fixation method has comparable strength to other fixation methods.[31]

When comparing unicortical button fixation and interference screw fixation, interference screw fixation has equivalent if not better pullout strength and displacement. Arora and colleagues[32] cautioned against using bicortical buttons due to the proximity of the axillary nerve; at the same time, they found the pullout strength similar between the unicortical button and interference screw. The senior author's study showed better ultimate failure load with the interference screw compared with the unicortical button; in addition, there was no added biomechanical benefit of using the interference screw in conjunction with a button.[33]

Another advantage of the subpectoral biceps tenodesis is the avoidance of over-tensioning. In a cadaveric study of 18 matched specimens, shoulders were randomized into subpectoral bicep tenodesis versus arthroscopic suprapectoral tenodesis.[34] Pretenodesis, a metallic bead was placed in the biceps tendon and a fluoroscopic image was obtained. Post-tenodesis, an image was obtained to evaluate the location of the tenodesis and the metallic bead and determine tensioning. Biomechanical load-to-failure

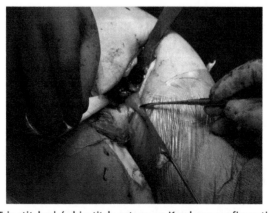

Fig. 10. The LHBT is stitched (whipstitch suture or Krackow configuration) starting 2 cm from the MTJ. The Freer elevator is demonstrating the starting position.

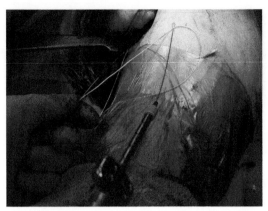

Fig. 11. By using a cannulated screwdriver, a lasso can be used to shuttle 1 of the sutures through the biceps tenodesis driver. The other suture is left free.

testing was then performed. The arthroscopic suprapectoral technique resulted in a significant 2-cm over-tensioning compared with the subpectoral technique. The arthroscopic suprapectoral technique also had significantly decreased ultimate load to failure compared with an open subpectoral technique in matched cadaveric specimens.

The depth and position of the interference screw have also been studied. In a study comparing tenodesis screw placed in the 50% proud, flush, or recessed position, the screws placed in the flush position had the highest ultimate load; however, this did not reach statistical significance.[35] In a study of 10 matched pairs of human humeri, subpectoral biceps tenodesis was evaluated with regard to the concentric position in the bicipital groove versus an eccentric position (30% to the lateral aspect of the humerus). Contralateral humeri remained intact as controls. Specimens were aligned in 40° of abduction, and a uniaxial compressive force was applied to the humeral head until failure. The eccentric humeral specimens had a significantly lower failure strength compared with controls, whereas the concentric humeral specimens were similar to controls. Laterally eccentric, malpositioned biceps tenodesis caused significant reduction (25%) in humeral strength, which may

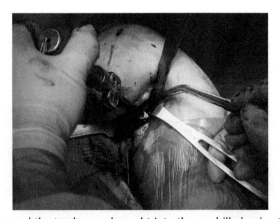

Fig. 12. The screw and the tendon are brought into the predrilled unicortical hole.

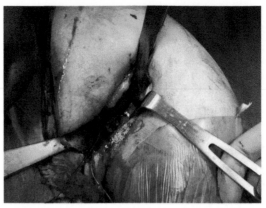

Fig. 13. The surgeon visually examines and palpates the tenodesis to confirm that the screw is flush with the cortex. The 2 ends of the suture are tied over the screw, securing the screw in place. The tendon often rotates in the tunnel to cover the screw, which is acceptable.

be clinically relevant and contribute to postsurgical humeral fracture. The investigators concluded that humeral fracture after subpectoral tenodesis of the LHBT is a complication that may be minimized with careful surgical technique using a centrally placed tenodesis site.

The previously described studies in cadaveric models all measure fixation strength at time zero. Thus, in vivo models are necessary to assess biomechanical strength of each method as the tenodesis site heals. Kilicoglu and colleagues[36] compared fixation in a sheep model using 3 fixation methods—suture sling through a bone tunnel, interference screw fixation, and suture anchors—in a time-dependent manner. On the day of implantation, the interference screw was the weakest construct in terms of maximum pullout strength. At 3 weeks, however, the interference screw had a higher mean ultimate load to failure compared with the other 2 methods of fixation, but this was not statistically significant. Additionally, the mean failure load was statistically significantly higher at 3 weeks than on the day of insertion for the interference screw.

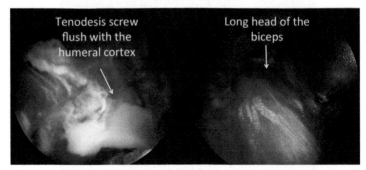

Fig. 14. Arthroscopic view of the flush tenodesis screw (*left*) and the insertion of the LHBT (*right*).

COMPLICATIONS AND MANAGEMENT

Recent literature also demonstrates major complications with subpectoral biceps tenodesis. A report of 4 cases by Rhee and colleagues[37] revealed iatrogenic brachial plexus injuries with the bicortical technique. In another case report, Sears and colleagues[38] demonstrated the risk of humeral fracture after subpectoral tenodesis in healthy patients. They recommend a precise strategy when choosing the operative technique and emphasize cautious postoperative activity limitations to reduce stress at the tenodesis site. This is further supported by Hipp and colleagues,[39] who showed in a finite element model reduced torsional strength by up to 60% when a hole with a diameter of 50% of the outer bone diameter is drilled. By combining these data to the mean humeral diameter of 18 mm to 21 mm,[40] Sears and colleagues[38] concluded that a cortical defect of approximately 8 mm would diminish bone strength. Furthermore, Euler and colleagues[41] conducted a biomechanical study investigating the optimal screw position by comparing concentrically and eccentrically placed tenodesis with regard to the bicipital groove. The results showed a significant reduction in humeral strength with eccentric screw postitioning. Thus, surgeons should always strive to optimize tunnel size and position when using a subpectoral biceps tenodesis technique.

POSTOPERATIVE CARE

Postoperative management depends on the type of treatment and is often limited due to additional surgery (eg, rotator cuff repair). If a subpectoral biceps tenodesis is the only treatment, no specific aftercare is required, beginning with passive range-of-motion exercises with progression to active assisted and active range of motion of the glenohumeral joint.[42] The authors recommend limited weight bearing for the first 12 weeks. Full elbow range of motion is allowed immediately. Braun and colleagues[6] recommend a sling until the wound is healed, with further limitations dictated by concomitant procedures.

CLINICAL OUTCOMES

With regard to clinical outcomes of open subpectoral tenodesis of the LHBT, good results have been reported. Mazzocca and colleagues[11] reported on 41 patients at an average follow-up of 29 months. None of these patient reported intertubercular groove pain. Among this cohort, 93% had no pain in the subpectoral triangle and 78% had no pain in the anterior aspect of the humerus. The mean pain score on the visual analog scale for the remaining was 1.1 (subpectoral triangle) and 1.8 (anterior humerus). In addition, Werner and colleagues[43] compared arthroscopic suprapectoral and open subpectoral biceps tenodesis and demonstrated excellent clinical and functional results for both techniques. After a mean follow-up of 3.1 years in 82 patients, no statistically significant difference in clinical outcomes could be identified. The arthroscopic group did, however, show a slightly increased rate of stiffness and overall total complication rate. These findings mirror the results of the same investigator,[44] who compared the 2 procedures in a group of 249 patients and found a statistically significant increased rate of postoperative stiffness (17.9%) in the arthroscopic group versus the open group (5.6%). This complication occurs more frequently in female patients, smokers, and with a more proximal tenodesis.[44,45] Nho and colleagues[46] demonstrated an overall complication rate of 2% in a population of 353 patients over the course of 3 years undergoing open subpectoral biceps tenodesis. Furthermore, Osbahr and colleagues[47] found more favorable cosmetic outcomes for biceps tenodesis compared with tenotomy. Although these outcomes are encouraging, no specific subpectoral technique has proved superior to the others, and more clinical studies are needed to provide more evidence.

REFERENCES

1. Gilcreest E. Two cases of spontaneous rupture of the long head of the biceps flexor cubiti. Surg Clin North Am 1926;6:539–54.
2. Boileau P, Neyton L. Arthroscopic tenodesis for lesions of the long head of the biceps. Oper Orthop Traumatol 2005;17(6):601–23.
3. Mazzocca AD, McCarthy MB, Ledgard FA, et al. Histomorphologic changes of the long head of the biceps tendon in common shoulder pathologies. Arthroscopy 2013;29(6):972–81.
4. Alpantaki K, McLaughlin D, Karagogeos D, et al. Sympathetic and sensory neural elements in the tendon of the long head of the biceps. J Bone Joint Surg Am 2005;87(7):1580–3.
5. Creech MJ, Yeung M, Denkers M, et al. Surgical indications for long head biceps tenodesis: a systematic review. Knee Surg Sports Traumatol Arthrosc 2014. [Epub ahead of print].
6. Braun S, Minzlaff P, Imhoff AB. Subpectoral tenodesis of the long head of the biceps tendon for pathologies of the long head of the biceps tendon and the biceps pulley. Oper Orthop Traumatol 2012;24(6):479–85 [in German].
7. Boileau P, Parratte S, Chuinard C, et al. Arthroscopic treatment of isolated type II SLAP lesions: biceps tenodesis as an alternative to reinsertion. Am J Sports Med 2009;37(5):929–36.
8. Sethi N, Wright R, Yamaguchi K. Disorders of the long head of the biceps tendon. J Shoulder Elbow Surg 1999;8(6):644–54.
9. Beitzel K, Mazzocca AD, Arciero RA. Clinical anatomy, biomechanics, physiologic function, history, examination, and radiographic evaluation of the biceps. Oper Tech Sports Med 2012;20(3):233–7.
10. Boileau P, Ahrens PM, Hatzidakis AM. Entrapment of the long head of the biceps tendon: the hourglass biceps–a cause of pain and locking of the shoulder. J Shoulder Elbow Surg 2004;13(3):249–57.
11. Mazzocca AD, Cote MP, Arciero CL, et al. Clinical outcomes after subpectoral biceps tenodesis with an interference screw. Am J Sports Med 2008;36(10):1922–9.
12. Snyder SJ. Shoulder arthroscopy. New York: McGraw-Hill; 1994.
13. Said HG, Babaqi AA, Mohamadean A, et al. Modified subpectoral biceps tenodesis. Int Orthop 2014;38(5):1063–6.
14. Kane P, Hsaio P, Tucker B, et al. Open subpectoral biceps tenodesis: reliable treatment for all biceps tendon pathology. Orthopedics 2015;38(1):37–41.
15. Snir N, Hamula M, Wolfson T, et al. Long head of the biceps tenodesis with cortical button technique. Arthrosc Tech 2013;2(2):e95–7.
16. Froimson AI, O I. Keyhole tenodesis of biceps origin at the shoulder. Clin Orthop Relat Res 1975;(112):245–9.
17. Reiff SN, Nho SJ, Romeo AA. Proximal humerus fracture after keyhole biceps tenodesis. Am J Orthop 2010;39(7):E61–3.
18. Amaravathi RS, Pankappilly B, Kany J. Arthroscopic keyhole proximal biceps tenodesis: a technical note. J Orthop Surg 2011;19(3):379–83.
19. Kany J, Guinand R, Amaravathi RS, et al. The keyhole technique for arthroscopic tenodesis of the long head of the biceps tendon. In vivo prospective study with a radio-opaque marker. Orthop Traumatol Surg Res 2015;101(1):31–4.
20. [abstract]. In: Sanders BS, Warner JP, Pennington S, editors. Biceps tendon tenodesis: success with proximal versus distal fixation. AAOS; 2007. Annual meeting proceedings.

21. Scully WF, Wilson DJ, Grassbaugh JA, et al. A simple surgical technique for sub-pectoral biceps tenodesis using a double-loaded suture anchor. Arthrosc Tech 2013;2(2):e191–6.
22. Su WR, Ling FY, Hong CK, et al. Subpectoral biceps tenodesis: a new technique using an all-suture anchor fixation. Knee Surg Sports Traumatol Arthrosc 2015; 23(2):596–9.
23. Mazzocca AD, Rios CG, Romeo AA, et al. Subpectoral biceps tenodesis with interference screw fixation. Arthroscopy 2005;21(7):896.
24. LaFrance R, Madsen W, Yaseen Z, et al. Relevant anatomic landmarks and mea-surements for biceps tenodesis. Am J Sports Med 2013;41(6):1395–9.
25. Sethi PM, Vadasdi K, Greene RT, et al. Safety of open suprapectoral and subpec-toral biceps tenodesis: an anatomic assessment of risk for neurologic injury. J Shoulder Elbow Surg 2015;24(1):138–42.
26. Dickens JF, Kilcoyne KG, Tintle SM, et al. Subpectoral biceps tenodesis: an anatomic study and evaluation of at-risk structures. Am J Sports Med 2012; 40(10):2337–41.
27. Carey P, Owens BD. Insertional footprint anatomy of the pectoralis major tendon. Orthopedics 2010;33(1):23.
28. Patzer T, Santo G, Olender GD, et al. Suprapectoral or subpectoral position for biceps tenodesis: biomechanical comparison of four different techniques in both positions. J Shoulder Elbow Surg 2012;21(1):116–25.
29. Tashjian RZ, Henninger HB. Biomechanical evaluation of subpectoral biceps te-nodesis: dual suture anchor versus interference screw fixation. J Shoulder Elbow Surg 2013;22(10):1408–12.
30. Richards DP, Burkhart SS. A biomechanical analysis of two biceps tenodesis fix-ation techniques. Arthroscopy 2005;21(7):861–6.
31. Mazzocca AD, Bicos J, Santangelo S, et al. The biomechanical evaluation of four fixation techniques for proximal biceps tenodesis. Arthroscopy 2005;21(11): 1296–306.
32. Arora AS, Singh A, Koonce RC. Biomechanical evaluation of a unicortical button versus interference screw for subpectoral biceps tenodesis. Arthroscopy 2013; 29(4):638–44.
33. Sethi PM, Rajaram A, Beitzel K, et al. Biomechanical performance of subpectoral biceps tenodesis: a comparison of interference screw fixation, cortical button fixation, and interference screw diameter. J Shoulder Elbow Surg 2013;22(4): 451–7.
34. Werner BC, Lyons ML, Evans CL, et al. Arthroscopic suprapectoral and open subpectoral biceps tenodesis: a comparison of restoration of length-tension and mechanical strength between techniques. Arthroscopy 2015;31(4):620–7.
35. Salata MJ, Bailey JR, Bell R, et al. Effect of interference screw depth on fixation strength in biceps tenodesis. Arthroscopy 2014;30(1):11–5.
36. Kilicoglu O, Koyuncu O, Demirhan M, et al. Time-dependent changes in failure loads of 3 biceps tenodesis techniques: in vivo study in a sheep model. Am J Sports Med 2005;33(10):1536–44.
37. Rhee PC, Spinner RJ, Bishop AT, et al. Iatrogenic brachial plexus injuries associ-ated with open subpectoral biceps tenodesis: a report of 4 cases. Am J Sports Med 2013;41(9):2048–53.
38. Sears BW, Spencer EE, Getz CL. Humeral fracture following subpectoral biceps tenodesis in 2 active, healthy patients. J Shoulder Elbow Surg 2011;20(6):e7–11.
39. Hipp JA, Edgerton BC, An KN, et al. Structural consequences of transcortical holes in long bones loaded in torsion. J Biomech 1990;23(12):1261–8.

40. Murdoch AH, Mathias KJ, Smith FW. Measurement of the bony anatomy of the humerus using magnetic resonance imaging. Proc Inst Mech Eng H 2002;216(1): 31–5.
41. Euler SA, Smith SD, Williams BT, et al. Biomechanical analysis of subpectoral biceps tenodesis: effect of screw malpositioning on proximal humeral strength. Am J Sports Med 2015;43(1):69–74.
42. O'Malley M, Beitzel K, Mazzocca AD. Disorders of the rotator intervall: coracohumeral ligament and biceps tendon. In: Milano G, Grasso A, editors. Shoulder arthroscopy. London: Springer-Verlag; 2014. p. 319–27.
43. Werner BC, Evans CL, Holzgrefe RE, et al. Arthroscopic suprapectoral and open subpectoral biceps tenodesis: a comparison of minimum 2-year clinical outcomes. Am J Sports Med 2014;42(11):2583–90.
44. Werner BC, Pehlivan HC, Hart JM, et al. Increased incidence of postoperative stiffness after arthroscopic compared with open biceps tenodesis. Arthroscopy 2014;30(9):1075–84.
45. Friedman DJ, Dunn JC, Higgins LD, et al. Proximal biceps tendon: injuries and management. Sports Med Arthrosc 2008;16(3):162–9.
46. Nho SJ, Reiff SN, Verma NN, et al. Complications associated with subpectoral biceps tenodesis: low rates of incidence following surgery. J Shoulder Elbow Surg 2010;19(5):764–8.
47. Osbahr DC, Diamond AB, Speer KP. The cosmetic appearance of the biceps muscle after long-head tenotomy versus tenodesis. Arthroscopy 2002;18(5): 483–7.

Proximal Biceps Tendon and Rotator Cuff Tears

Mandeep S. Virk, MD[a], Brian J. Cole, MD, MBA[b],*

KEYWORDS

• Biceps tenotomy • Biceps tenodesis • Rotator cuff tears

KEY POINTS

• Long head of the biceps is commonly involved in rotator cuff tears.
• Both tenotomy and tenodesis are effective in relieving pain from biceps tendon disorder in the presence of rotator cuff tears.
• Tenotomy of the proximal biceps is a safe and quick procedure, but can be associated with a clinically significant Popeye sign and cramps in the biceps muscle.
• Tenodesis of the LHBT establishes the length-tension relationship and minimizes the risk of Popeye deformity.

INTRODUCTION

The functional role of the long head of the biceps tendon (LHBT) in glenohumeral joint stability is poorly understood and remains controversial. From the anatomic perspective, the LHBT is fixed at its origin on the supraglenoid tubercle and the superior labrum.[1] With the shoulder in neutral or internal rotation, the LHBT courses in an oblique direction from its origin toward the intertubercular groove.[2] The tendon is stabilized by the medial sling, which is formed by the coracohumeral and superior glenohumeral ligaments.[3–5] The role of the transverse humeral ligament as a medial restraint is less established.[4] In external rotation and abduction of shoulder, the LHBT is prevented from posterior subluxation by the posterior sling formed by the posterior part of the coracohumeral ligament and the anterior fibers of the supraspinatus tendon.[2,6,7] This unique anatomy of the proximal biceps places it at high risk for abrasive wear and injury. Furthermore, its close proximity to the anterior and superior rotator cuff predisposes the LHBT to injury in the setting of rotator cuff tears.

[a] Division of Shoulder and Elbow Surgery, Department of Orthopaedic Surgery, NYU-Langone Medical Center, NYU-Hospital for Joint Diseases, 301 East 17th Street, New York, NY 10003, USA; [b] Division of Shoulder and Elbow and Sports Medicine, Department of Orthopaedic Surgery, Rush University Medical Center, 1611 West Harrison Street, Chicago, IL 60612, USA
* Corresponding author.
E-mail address: bcole@rushortho.com

Clin Sports Med 35 (2016) 153–161
http://dx.doi.org/10.1016/j.csm.2015.08.010   sportsmed.theclinics.com
0278-5919/16/$ – see front matter © 2016 Elsevier Inc. All rights reserved.

PROXIMAL BICEPS AND ROTATOR CUFF TEARS
Disorders

The LHBT lies in close anatomic proximity to the subscapularis and supraspinatus tendons. Rotator cuff tears have a high incidence of concomitant LHBT disorder, and this disorder is directly correlated with the extent of rotator cuff disease.[8,9] Tendon hypertrophy, hourglass contracture, delamination, partial and complete tears, and tendon instability in the bicipital groove are common macroscopic pathologic findings affecting the LHBT in the presence of rotator cuff tears (**Fig. 1**).[1,9–12] Early on in the rotator cuff degenerative process, LHBT disorder may present as purely microscopic or may show mild thickening of the intra-articular part of the tendon, synovitis, or dynamic subluxation. Some of these findings are more pronounced in the intertubercular part of the LHBT and can easily be missed during arthroscopy if the tendon is not pulled into the joint with a probe to examine the intertubercular part of the tendon.[13,14]

SPONTANEOUS RUPTURE OF THE LONG HEAD OF THE BICEPS TENDON

Spontaneous complete rupture of the LHBT can occur in the presence of chronic rotator cuff tears.[10] Usually the patient reports hearing a snap during a common activity or during mildly strenuous activity. Patients often report relief of shoulder pain

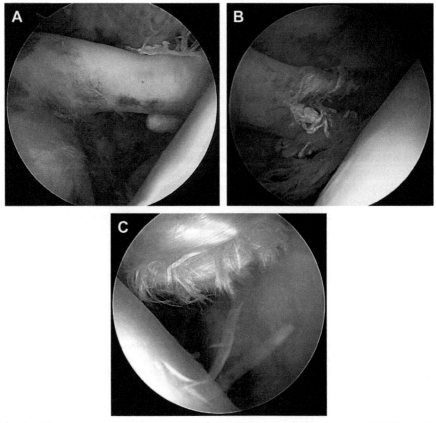

Fig. 1. Arthroscopic images (viewing from the posterior portal) showing synovitis (A), partial tear (B), and delamination (C) of the long head of the biceps concomitant with rotator cuff tear.

following complete ruptures.[15,16] Complete rupture of the LHBT can result in loss of normal arm contour caused by distal migration of the biceps muscle belly, which is popularly described as the Popeye sign. However, not all patients complain of a Popeye deformity or have biceps cramping following complete ruptures of the LHBT. Absence of a Popeye deformity after complete biceps rupture is thought to be caused by scarring of the tendon in the bicipital groove, rotator interval, or by the subscapularis tendon. In older patients, this deformity may be less noticeable because of muscle atrophy.[11]

MECHANICAL ENTRAPMENT OF THE DISEASED LONG HEAD OF THE BICEPS TENDON

In rotator cuff tears, the LHBT can be mechanically entrapped intra-articularly or in the bicipital groove. Boileau and colleagues[11] described the hourglass biceps, which is hypertrophy of the intra-articular portion of the LHBT, which then gets trapped in the joint during elevation of the arm, resulting in pain and restriction of shoulder elevation. The intertubercular portion of the LHBT can be scarred in this location because of synovial adhesions. In our experience performing open subpectoral biceps tenodesis, an LHBT that is scarred in the groove often does not drop after tenotomy, and often requires more force to retrieve during tenodesis. Furthermore, in these cases the retrieved tendon often shows synovial bands and inflammation.[17]

INSTABILITY OF THE LONG HEAD OF THE BICEPS TENDON

Medial instability of the LHBT is caused by failure of the medial sling of the biceps, which is composed of the superior glenohumeral ligament and the coracohumeral ligament.[18] Medial instability of the LHBT is characteristically seen with anterosuperior rotator cuff tears (subscapularis and supraspinatus). Walch and colleagues[18] reported a detailed description of instability of biceps tendon in association with rotator cuff tears. In their retrospective review of 446 shoulders with rotator cuff tears, they found instability in 71 cases. The LHBT was subluxated in 25 shoulders and dislocated in 46 shoulders. Dislocation of the LHBT was seen in association with complete tears of subscapularis in 23 cases, partial tears of subscapularis in 21 cases, and with an intact subscapularis in 2 cases. The tendon subluxation was either in the form of slippage along the superior part of the lesser tuberosity or over the medial rim of the groove. Medial dislocation of the LHBT was present in the form of intra-articular dislocation in 23 cases, dislocation into the substance of subscapularis in 21 cases, and over the intact subscapularis tendon in 2 cases. Note that the LHBT was fairly normal in appearance with minimal damage when the tendon was dislocated intra-articularly but had variable degrees of damage when the tendon was subluxated into the subscapularis. Although posterior dislocation of the LHBT is uncommon and is seen in association with acute posttraumatic posterosuperior rotator cuff tears, Lafosse and colleagues[6] reported a higher incidence of LHBT instability in a prospective series of 200 patients who underwent arthroscopic rotator cuff repair. The LHBT stability was tested statically and dynamically in the anterior-posterior direction during diagnostic shoulder arthroscopic examination. Instability of LHBT was present in 89 of 200 shoulders (45%) with the instability pattern of 37% in the anterior direction, 42% in the posterior direction, and 21% in both the anterior and posterior direction. Anterior instability of the LHBT was in the form of subluxation or dislocation of the tendon, but posterior and combined anterior and posterior instability was always a subluxation event, which was reducible.

DIAGNOSIS AND IMAGING

Proximal biceps (LHBT) disorder usually results in anterior shoulder pain with radiation into the arm along the muscle belly in some cases.[19,20] However, there is no discrete pain pattern or distribution that is specific to LHBT disorders. It may be difficult to isolate signs and symptoms specific to proximal biceps tendon disorder in the presence of rotator cuff disorder during physical examination. Although multiple physical examination signs and special tests have been described for the diagnosis of biceps tendon disorder in the setting of rotator cuff tears, there is no single test that is 100% sensitive and specific.[20,21] Tenderness to palpation directly over the upper part of the bicipital groove or in the subpectoral location is a sensitive test but lacks specificity. The Popeye sign is diagnostic of a drooping biceps but not all LHBT ruptures result in this deformity. An anteriorly dislocated LHBT can be palpated and rolled under the finger in thin individuals.

Plain radiographs are not helpful in the diagnosis of LHBT disorder. MRI, computed tomography arthrography, and ultrasonography are widely used but sensitivities are low.[22,23] Arthroscopic evaluation is considered the gold standard for evaluation of the LHBT.[22] It is critical to evaluate the intertubercular portion of the proximal biceps for signs of disorder (synovitis, dynamic instability) during diagnostic arthroscopy (**Fig. 2**).[14]

TREATMENT

Nonsurgical management of proximal biceps tendinopathy has traditionally included activity modification, physical therapy, antiinflammatory medications, and corticosteroid injections into the glenohumeral joint, subacromial space, or into the biceps tendon sheath in the groove.[14,24] Biceps tenotomy and biceps tenodesis are surgical treatment options for addressing LHBT disorder.[24]

Tenotomy of the LHBT relieves pain by preventing traction insult to the inflamed or degenerated biceps tendon (**Fig. 3**). Proponents of biceps tenotomy consider it a simple and safe procedure that consistently relieves pain and allows quicker

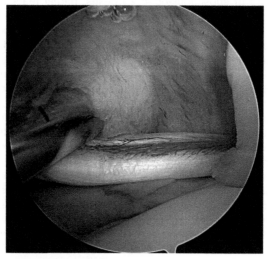

Fig. 2. Arthroscopic examination of the intertubercular portion of the long head of the biceps showing synovitis (lip stick lesion).

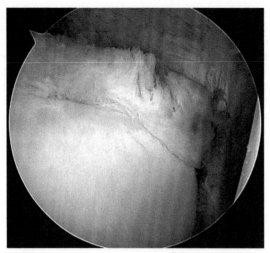

Fig. 3. Arthroscopic image (viewing from the posterior portal) of superior labrum after biceps tenotomy.

rehabilitation. Tenotomy of the LHBT can be associated with Popeye deformity and biceps cramping, which can result in poor satisfaction in young patients **(Fig. 4)**.[15,16,25,26] Biceps tenodesis provides a new fixation point for the tenotomized tendon in the proximal humerus, and thus maintains the length-tension relationship of the musculotendinous unit. However, the tenodesis has to be protected and requires an initial period of immobilization.[14,27–29] Patients who cannot comply with the initial period of immobilization and slower rehabilitation are more appropriately treated with tenotomy. Many surgical techniques have been described for arthroscopic and open biceps tenodesis and description is beyond the scope of this article. Debate remains regarding the ideal location, ideal implant, and ideal technique for biceps tenodesis.

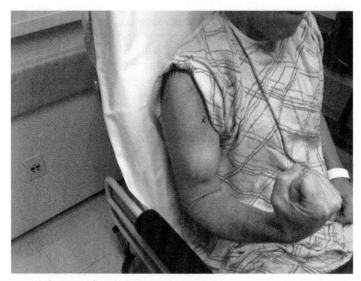

Fig. 4. Popeye deformity after arthroscopic tenotomy.

Failure to address LHBT disorder in the setting of rotator cuff repair can result in persistent shoulder pain and poor patient satisfaction. The role of biceps tenotomy or tenodesis as a treatment of LHBT disorder along with concomitant rotator cuff repair has been extensively studied.[15,16,27,30–34] In a prospective, randomized controlled study, Zhang and colleagues[34] reported no significant differences in the clinical results, outcome scores, cosmetic deformity, biceps cramping, and satisfaction level between arthroscopic biceps tenotomy and tenodesis in patients older than 55 years with reparable rotator cuff tears. In a prospective cohort study comparing biceps tenotomy with tenodesis in the setting of rotator cuff repairs, Koh and colleagues[27] reported a significantly higher rate of Popeye deformity and higher rate of biceps cramping with tenotomy. There were no differences between the two groups with respect to outcome scores (Constant and American Shoulder and Elbow Surgeons scores). De Carli and colleagues[31] reported similar findings in a retrospective study comparing arthroscopic tenotomy (n = 30) with arthroscopic tenodesis (n = 35) in patients with reparable rotator cuff tears and LHBT disorder. The investigators found no significant differences between the two groups with respect to pain relief and functional outcome. A recent meta-analysis by Leroux and colleagues[33] comparing outcomes after biceps tenotomy or tenodesis performed with rotator cuff repair showed significant improvement in postoperative Constant scores. However, the difference in Constant scores between the two groups was lower than the reported minimal clinically important difference. Similarly, biceps deformity was significantly less in the tenodesis group compared with the tenotomy group but most of the patients were not concerned with the cosmetic deformity. There was no significant difference between the two groups with respect to satisfaction rate and rate of biceps cramping.

Tenotomy of the LHBT in massive rotator cuff tears was first proposed by Gilles Walch to relieve pain and improve function (see **Fig. 3**). In a retrospective case series, Walch and colleagues[16] reported their long-term results of arthroscopic tenotomy in 307 cases with an average follow-up of 57 months (range, 24–168 months). Arthroscopic tenotomy was offered as a surgical treatment to patients with irreparable rotator cuff tears and to patients who were not willing to participate in the rehabilitation required after rotator cuff repair. There was a significant improvement in postoperative mean Constant scores and 87% of patients were satisfied or very satisfied with the result. The investigators described the biceps tenotomy as a purely palliative procedure, which does not protect against the progressive radiographic changes that occur with long-standing rotator cuff disease. Small retrospective case series have shown favorable results with arthroscopic biceps tenotomy for concomitant LHBT disorder in the presence of rotator cuff tears. In another retrospective case study, Boileau and colleagues[15] compared arthroscopic biceps tenotomy (n = 39) with biceps tenodesis (n = 33) for treatment of persistent shoulder pain and dysfunction caused by irreparable rotator cuff tears with proximal biceps lesion. Postoperatively, there was significant improvement in the mean Constant score and 78% of the patients were satisfied with the procedure. There were no significant differences between the tenotomy and tenodesis groups with satisfaction rate and mean Constant scores. Sixty-two percent of the shoulders in the tenotomy group had a Popeye sign, although none were bothered by it.

The aforementioned studies show that biceps tenotomy and biceps tenodesis are both effective treatment options for addressing LHBT disorder in the setting of rotator cuff tears. Cosmetic deformity, muscle cramps, and strength deficits are three of the most common adverse events associated with biceps tenotomy. The incidence of biceps cramping, and concern regarding cosmetic deformity, are less pronounced in the elderly patient population and these conditions seldom require revision surgery.

However, cosmetic concerns can be important in young, thin patients. Further, loss of elbow strength, especially supination strength, may result in poor satisfaction in manual laborers. Compared with the biceps tenotomy, the advantages of tenodesis include less risk of postoperative cramping and an improved cosmetic result. However, biceps tenodesis is a more complex operation that requires a period of postoperative immobilization and lengthier rehabilitation.

As per the senior author's protocol, we maintain a low threshold to treat the biceps tendon in the setting of a surgically managed rotator cuff tear. Any pathologic abnormalities of the tendon generally lead to concomitant treatment of the biceps, especially in a revision setting or following occupational injuries in an effort to eradicate all potential pain generators. We prefer to perform biceps tenodesis in young and active patients, patients with heavy physical recreational or occupational demands, and thin muscular patients. Biceps tenotomy is reserved for the older patient population with sedentary demands, in situations in which cosmesis is not a concern, and in patients who cannot comply with the initial protective rehabilitation protocol.

SUMMARY

The LHBT lies in the rotator interval between the subscapularis and supraspinatus tendons and is commonly pathologic in the setting of rotator cuff tears. Failure to address LHBT disorder in reparable rotator cuff tears can result in residual postoperative pain and poor outcomes. There is controversy regarding whether biceps tenotomy or tenodesis is superior for surgical treatment of biceps disorder in the setting of rotator cuff tears. Tenotomy is a simple, quick, and safe procedure, but carries a risk of biceps cramping and deformity. Tenodesis restores the length-tension relationship of the biceps and minimizes the risk of biceps cramping and Popeye deformity. However, comparative retrospective studies do not show any significant improvement in shoulder outcome measures and pain relief with biceps tenodesis compared with tenotomy in the setting of rotator cuff tears.

REFERENCES

1. Refior HJ, Sowa D. Long tendon of the biceps brachii: sites of predilection for degenerative lesions. J Shoulder Elbow Surg 1995;4:436–40.
2. Sethi N, Wright R, Yamaguchi K. Disorders of the long head of the biceps tendon. J Shoulder Elbow Surg 1999;8:644–54.
3. Bennett WF. Visualization of the anatomy of the rotator interval and bicipital sheath. Arthroscopy 2001;17:107–11.
4. Kwon YW, Hurd J, Yeager K, et al. Proximal biceps tendon–a biomechanical analysis of the stability at the bicipital groove. Bull NYU Hosp Jt Dis 2009;67:337–40.
5. Arai R, Mochizuki T, Yamaguchi K, et al. Functional anatomy of the superior glenohumeral and coracohumeral ligaments and the subscapularis tendon in view of stabilization of the long head of the biceps tendon. J Shoulder Elbow Surg 2010;19:58–64.
6. Lafosse L, Reiland Y, Baier GP, et al. Anterior and posterior instability of the long head of the biceps tendon in rotator cuff tears: a new classification based on arthroscopic observations. Arthroscopy 2007;23:73–80.
7. Habermeyer P, Magosch P, Pritsch M, et al. Anterosuperior impingement of the shoulder as a result of pulley lesions: a prospective arthroscopic study. J Shoulder Elbow Surg 2004;13:5–12.

8. Murthi AM, Vosburgh CL, Neviaser TJ. The incidence of pathologic changes of the long head of the biceps tendon. J Shoulder Elbow Surg 2000;9:382–5.

9. Chen CH, Hsu KY, Chen WJ, et al. Incidence and severity of biceps long head tendon lesion in patients with complete rotator cuff tears. J Trauma 2005;58:1189–93.

10. Ahrens PM, Boileau P. The long head of biceps and associated tendinopathy. J Bone Joint Surg Br 2007;89:1001–9.

11. Boileau P, Ahrens PM, Hatzidakis AM. Entrapment of the long head of the biceps tendon: the hourglass biceps–a cause of pain and locking of the shoulder. J Shoulder Elbow Surg 2004;13:249–57.

12. Sakurai G, Ozaki J, Tomita Y, et al. Morphologic changes in long head of biceps brachii in rotator cuff dysfunction. J Orthop Sci 1998;3:137–42.

13. Mazzocca AD, McCarthy MB, Ledgard FA, et al. Histomorphologic changes of the long head of the biceps tendon in common shoulder pathologies. Arthroscopy 2013;29:972–81.

14. Nho SJ, Strauss EJ, Lenart BA, et al. Long head of the biceps tendinopathy: diagnosis and management. J Am Acad Orthop Surg 2010;18:645–56.

15. Boileau P, Baque F, Valerio L, et al. Isolated arthroscopic biceps tenotomy or tenodesis improves symptoms in patients with massive irreparable rotator cuff tears. J Bone Joint Surg Am 2007;89:747–57.

16. Walch G, Edwards TB, Boulahia A, et al. Arthroscopic tenotomy of the long head of the biceps in the treatment of rotator cuff tears: clinical and radiographic results of 307 cases. J Shoulder Elbow Surg 2005;14:238–46.

17. Singaraju VM, Kang RW, Yanke AB, et al. Biceps tendinitis in chronic rotator cuff tears: a histologic perspective. J Shoulder Elbow Surg 2008;17:898–904.

18. Walch G, Nove-Josserand L, Boileau P, et al. Subluxations and dislocations of the tendon of the long head of the biceps. J Shoulder Elbow Surg 1998;7:100–8.

19. Szabo I, Boileau P, Walch G. The proximal biceps as a pain generator and results of tenotomy. Sports Med Arthrosc 2008;16:180–6.

20. Hegedus EJ, Goode AP, Cook CE, et al. Which physical examination tests provide clinicians with the most value when examining the shoulder? Update of a systematic review with meta-analysis of individual tests. Br J Sports Med 2012; 46:964–78.

21. Ben Kibler W, Sciascia AD, Hester P, et al. Clinical utility of traditional and new tests in the diagnosis of biceps tendon injuries and superior labrum anterior and posterior lesions in the shoulder. Am J Sports Med 2009;37:1840–7.

22. Dubrow SA, Streit JJ, Shishani Y, et al. Diagnostic accuracy in detecting tears in the proximal biceps tendon using standard nonenhancing shoulder MRI. Open Access J Sports Med 2014;5:81–7.

23. Skendzel JG, Jacobson JA, Carpenter JE, et al. Long head of biceps brachii tendon evaluation: accuracy of preoperative ultrasound. AJR Am J Roentgenol 2011;197:942–8.

24. Khazzam M, George MS, Churchill RS, et al. Disorders of the long head of biceps tendon. J Shoulder Elbow Surg 2012;21:136–45.

25. Duff SJ, Campbell PT. Patient acceptance of long head of biceps brachii tenotomy. J Shoulder Elbow Surg 2012;21:61–5.

26. Kelly AM, Drakos MC, Fealy S, et al. Arthroscopic release of the long head of the biceps tendon: functional outcome and clinical results. Am J Sports Med 2005; 33:208–13.

27. Koh KH, Ahn JH, Kim SM, et al. Treatment of biceps tendon lesions in the setting of rotator cuff tears: prospective cohort study of tenotomy versus tenodesis. Am J Sports Med 2010;38:1584–90.

28. Mazzocca AD, Cote MP, Arciero CL, et al. Clinical outcomes after subpectoral biceps tenodesis with an interference screw. Am J Sports Med 2008;36:1922–9.
29. Slenker NR, Lawson K, Ciccotti MG, et al. Biceps tenotomy versus tenodesis: clinical outcomes. Arthroscopy 2012;28:576–82.
30. Biz C, Vinanti GB, Rossato A, et al. Prospective study of three surgical procedures for long head biceps tendinopathy associated with rotator cuff tears. Muscles Ligaments Tendons J 2012;2:133–6.
31. De Carli A, Vadala A, Zanzotto E, et al. Reparable rotator cuff tears with concomitant long-head biceps lesions: tenotomy or tenotomy/tenodesis? Knee Surg Sports Traumatol Arthrosc 2012;20:2553–8.
32. Kukkonen J, Rantakokko J, Virolainen P, et al. The effect of biceps procedure on the outcome of rotator cuff reconstruction. ISRN Orthop 2013;2013:840965.
33. Leroux T, Chahal J, Wasserstein D, et al. A systematic review and meta-analysis comparing clinical outcomes after concurrent rotator cuff repair and long head biceps tenodesis or tenotomy. Sports Health 2015;7:303–7.
34. Zhang Q, Zhou J, Ge H, et al. Tenotomy or tenodesis for long head biceps lesions in shoulders with reparable rotator cuff tears: a prospective randomised trial. Knee Surg Sports Traumatol Arthrosc 2015;23:464–9.

Proximal Biceps in Overhead Athletes

Peter N. Chalmers, MD*, Nikhil N. Verma, MD

KEYWORDS

- Biceps tendonitis • Overhead athletes • Baseball • SLAP tear

KEY POINTS

- Proximal biceps disorder is a common cause of pain and dysfunction in overhead athletes, particularly pitchers.
- Diagnosis of bicipital tendonitis is driven by tenderness to palpation, but can be challenging for superior labral anterior-posterior (SLAP) tears.
- Diagnostic imaging with MRI can be difficult to interpret secondary to high rates of false positives.
- Nonoperative treatment with nonsteroidal anti-inflammatory medications, targeted ultrasound-guided corticosteroid injections, and supervised physical therapy focusing on rotator cuff strengthening, scapular stabilization, and scapular dyskinesis is indicated as the first-line option in all cases.
- For operative treatment the options include SLAP repair (for SLAP tears) and biceps tenodesis (for both SLAP tears and bicipital tendonitis). Return to play can be unpredictable after SLAP repair. Biceps tenodesis has consistent and reliable results, but limited data exist regarding return to play.

INTRODUCTION

The proximal tendon of the long head of the biceps (LHBT) has an anatomically unique course, passing lateral to the lesser tuberosity in the intertubercular groove before turning 30° medially and posteriorly to pass into the glenohumeral joint and to insert on the superior labrum and supraglenoid tubercle.[1] A spectrum of pathologic

The work for this article was performed at Rush University Medical Center in Chicago, IL.
Disclosures: Dr P.N. Chalmers has nothing to disclose. Dr N.N. Verma receives royalties from Smith & Nephew, is a pain consultant for MinInvasive and Smith & Nephew; has stock or stock options in Cymedica, minInvasive, and Omeros; receives research support from Arthrex, Smith & Nephew, Athletico, ConMed Linvatec, Miomed, Mitek, Arthrosurface, and DJ Orthopedics; receives publishing royalties from Vindico Medical-Orthopedics Hyperguide and Arthroscopy; serves on boards or committees for Journal of Knee Surgery, Arthroscopy, SLACK Incorporated, and the Arthroscopy Association Learning Center Committee.
Department of Orthopaedic Surgery, Rush University Medical Center, 1611 West Harrison Street, Suite 200, Chicago, IL 60612, USA
* Corresponding author.
E-mail address: p.n.chalmers@gmail.com

Clin Sports Med 35 (2016) 163–179
http://dx.doi.org/10.1016/j.csm.2015.08.009
0278-5919/16/$ – see front matter © 2016 Elsevier Inc. All rights reserved.

conditions can occur along this course, ranging from bicipital tendonitis, to bicipital instability, to lesions of the LHBT pulley, to superior labral anterior-posterior (SLAP) tears.[1,2] SLAP tears were originally described by Andrews and colleagues[3] in 1985, and have been classified by Snyder and coleagues.[4] More than 50% of these tears are type II tears whereby the LHBT anchor and labrum are torn and detached from the glenoid rim.[4] SLAP tears and bicipital tendonitis can occur with partial-thickness articular-sided posterosuperior rotator cuff tears in the setting of internal impingement, anteroinferior labral tears in the setting of glenohumeral instability, or a variety of other disorders, so a thorough assessment is necessary. Disorders of the LHBT are commonly encountered, with SLAP tears being found in up to 26% of shoulder arthroscopies.[5] In addition, operative treatment of SLAP tears is common and seems to be increasing, currently accounting for 10% of shoulder surgeries among recent residency graduates.[6,7] Biceps tenodesis also appears to be increasing: a recent large database study reported a 1.7-fold increase in its incidence between 2008 and 2011.[8]

Injuries to the superior labrum-long head biceps complex are commonly encountered in 2 patient groups: those that occur among young athletes and those that occur within older overhead manual laborers.[4] Among athletes, the sporting activities most commonly affected include baseball pitching, softball, tennis, swimming, volleyball, and other overhead sporting activities.[9] Baseball pitching is particularly associated with SLAP tears. The overhand baseball pitch is one of the fastest human motions, with humeral angular velocities exceeding 7000° per second.[10] During this motion enormous forces are placed on the shoulder, regularly exceeding 1000 N in professional pitchers just after ball release.[10] These forces are greater than 4 times the forces within the kicking leg.[11] To produce high-velocity pitches, the arm undergoes a series of compensatory changes, including increased external rotation and decreased internal rotation through ligamentous, muscular, and osseous remodeling.[9]

The baseball pitch is divided into 6 phases: wind-up, stride, cocking, acceleration, deceleration, and follow-through (**Fig. 1**). This motion is a kinetic chain whereby energy is created in the large muscles of the lower extremity and core, and then transferred through the shoulder and elbow onto the ball.[12] During the wind-up and stride phases, the pitcher brings the lead leg into hip and knee flexion and then strides downhill on the mound toward the plate while rotating the pelvis to face home plate and moving the arm to reach the "slot" position, where the shoulder, elbow, and hand are coplanar with both shoulders roughly at front foot strike. During the cocking phase, the shoulders rotate to be parallel with the pelvis while the shoulder "cocks" into maximal external rotation. During acceleration the arm then accelerates into internal rotation while the elbow extends. During this phase the pitcher imparts angular moment of the ball through motion of the forearm and specialized ball grips to create breaking pitches. Once the arm has reached maximal velocity, the ball is released and the deceleration phase begins. During this phase large distraction forces occur within the shoulder and there is a decelerating external rotation torque.[10]

Several portions of the overhand pitch may be associated with SLAP tears, and the pathologic etiology remains controversial. Some investigators have theorized that during the deceleration and follow-through phase the LHBT is maximally tensioned and that these distractive forces in line with the LHBT across the internally rotated glenohumeral joint may lift the labrum and LHBT anchor from the glenoid rim.[3,13] Others have theorized that during the late cocking phase, the arm is maximally abducted and externally rotated and, thus, the vertical, posteriorly directed LHBT tendon may "peel back" from the glenoid rim.[14] This phenomenon can be observed arthroscopically (**Fig. 2**).[14–16] These 2 competing theories have also been combined into the "weed-pull" theory whereby the back-and-forth sawing motion of the high-velocity

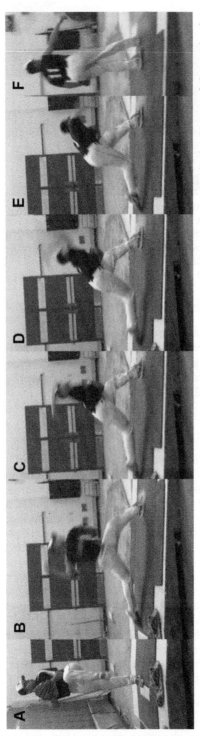

Fig. 1. Phases of the pitch. The major events of the pitch are demonstrated. (A) Lead foot maximum elevation, the beginning of the stride phase. (B) Front foot stride, the beginning of the cocking phase. (C) Maximum external rotation, the beginning of the acceleration phase. (D) Ball release, the beginning of the deceleration phase. (E) Maximum internal rotation, the beginning of the follow-through phase. (F) Lag foot strike, the end of the follow-through phase.

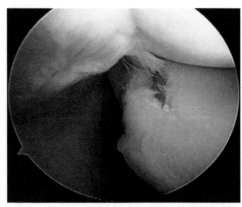

Fig. 2. Arthroscopic image of the right shoulder in the lateral decubitus position viewed from posteriorly demonstrates "peel-back" of a superior labral anterior-posterior tear. The patient's arm is being abducted and externally rotated into the "cocking" position. The internal impingement between the posterosuperior rotator cuff, which demonstrates mild fraying, and the posterosuperior glenoid can also be observed in this position. The biceps tendon can be seen in the middle of the image.

overhand pitch between external rotation in cocking and internal rotation in follow-through may pull the LHBT anchor from the glenoid rim.[17] Associated disorders such as anterior microinstability and posterior capsular contracture may also play a role.[3,17] Just as the etiology of SLAP tears is not well agreed upon, treatment of these lesions remains a source of significant controversy among surgeons and within the literature. Of note, SLAP tears may not be pathologic in baseball players: in a recent review of shoulder MRI in 21 asymptomatic professional pitchers, 10 had SLAP tears.[18]

OVERVIEW OF PATIENT EVALUATION

As with other conditions of the shoulder, evaluation of lesions of the proximal biceps tendon requires a full history. Although microtrauma caused by repetitive activities is the most common mechanism of injury,[1] more acute traumatic mechanisms are possible. In general, patients complain of anterolateral shoulder pain radiating down the biceps muscle exacerbated by overhead athletic activities such as throwing or overhead lifting.[2] The LHBT is densely innervated with pain fibers, so disorders of the proximal biceps can be painful.[19] SLAP tears may result in pain in a more posterior-superior position. In particular, baseball pitchers may have pain during the late cocking phase,[20] whereas tennis players may suffer pain during the cocking stage of the serve.[21] Patients with instability of the biceps tendon may experience mechanical clicking, popping, or audible snapping.[2] Unstable SLAP tears may manifest similar mechanical symptoms, although this is less common.[20] Concomitant anomalies are common with biceps tendonitis and SLAP tears: the symptoms of concomitant rotator cuff tears,[22] subacromial impingement, anterior capsular disorder, glenohumeral chondral defects, and other pathologic conditions may obscure or overlap with those symptoms generated by the biceps tendon.[1]

Physical Examination Maneuvers

Several physical examination findings are associated with disorders of the proximal biceps tendon. After a full general shoulder examination including inspection, palpation, range of motion, rotator cuff and deltoid strength testing, and distal neurovascular testing, specific provocative maneuvers are performed. For bicipital tendonitis the most common physical examination test is tenderness to palpation at the bicipital groove, which can be palpated both proximal and distal to the pectoralis tendon with the arm in slight internal rotation 2 to 3 inches (5–7.5 cm) distal to the acromion. Medial and lateral movement of the tenderness with internal and external rotation of the shoulder is also confirmatory.[2] The Speed maneuver (pain with resisted elbow flexion)[23] and the Yergason maneuver (pain with resisted forearm supination)[2] have been described traditionally, although the authors have not found these tests to be clinically useful. For SLAP tears a wide variety of physical examination maneuvers have been described, which speaks to the difficulty of diagnosing this lesion on physical examination. Examples include the active compression test,[24] the passive compression test,[25] the anterior slide test,[26] the crank test,[27] the Mayo dynamic shear test,[28] and the SLAPrehension test.[29] Biceps tendon instability is associated with subscapularis tears, which may demonstrate positive lift-off, belly-press, or internal rotation lag signs.[29] Finally, rotational range of motion at the shoulder should be evaluated. To accurately evaluate shoulder rotational range of motion, the patient should lie supine on the examination table while the examiner stabilizes the scapula by pressing against the coracoid and acromion. The shoulder is then rotated until the scapula can be felt to rotate under the stabilizing hand. Range of motion can then be tested with a goniometer looking from the lateral aspect of the shoulder. Accurate measurement of bilateral shoulder rotational range of motion is critical in identifying subtle loss of total range of motion or glenohumeral internal rotation deficit (GIRD).

Diagnostic Imaging

Patients should first be evaluated with a complete shoulder series, including Grashey anteroposterior, scapular-Y lateral, and axillary lateral radiographs, to rule out concomitant osseous disorder. However, in most patients proximal biceps tendon disorders cannot be visualized on plain radiographs, and MRI is necessary. On MRI the most typical finding of an SLAP tear is a cleft between the glenoid and the superior labrum (**Fig. 3**). However, wide anatomic variation exists within the anterosuperior

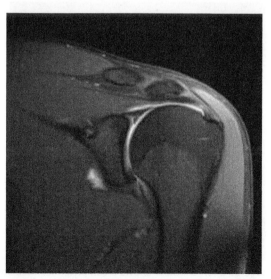

Fig. 3. Coronal MR image of a left shoulder shows a superior labral anterior-posterior tear.

labrum. For instance, the superior labrum may have a meniscoid quality with a cleft between the articular cartilage and the labrum itself. The anterosuperior labrum may have an anatomic sublabral foramen, or the middle glenohumeral ligament may attach at the anterosuperior labrum, in what has been termed the Buford complex.[30] Associated findings can include cysts (**Fig. 4**), which can compress the suprascapular nerve at the spinoglenoid notch, leading to isolated infraspinatus weakness.[31] In cases of bicipital tendonitis, increased fluid surrounding the tendon can be observed. In addition, the tendon can develop longitudinal split tears, especially in association with subscapularis tears and bicipital tendon instability (**Fig. 5**). SLAP tears are notoriously difficult to diagnose on MRI images: in one recent study the accuracy of MRI was 76%, the positive predictive value was 24%, and the negative predictive value was 95%. Adding intra-articular gadolinium for a magnetic resonance arthrogram (MRA) slightly improves sensitivity from 66% to 80% and improves positive predictive value to 29%, but increases the false-positive rate and thus decreases overall accuracy to 69%.[32] MRI has been demonstrated to be accurate for biceps pulley lesions.[33] Ultrasonography is an emerging imaging modality for the diagnosis of biceps tendon disorder, although it has not yet achieved widespread use and does not allow evaluation of the biceps anchor, and thus provides only limited information.[34] In all cases, diagnostic imaging must be correlated with patient history and clinical examination findings to establish a working diagnosis.

PHARMACOLOGIC TREATMENT OPTIONS

Because proximal biceps tendon abnormalities in the athlete are inflammatory in etiology, anti-inflammatory medication with nonsteroidal anti-inflammatory medications, a pulse of systemic corticosteroids, localized corticosteroid injections, and localized nonsteroidal anti-inflammatory medication injections are usually attempted as first-line treatment. Whereas intra-articular injections have been given for SLAP tears, bicipital tendonitis often responds well to injection of the biceps sheath. Although

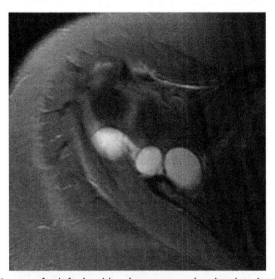

Fig. 4. Axial MR image of a left shoulder shows a complex, loculated spinoglenoid notch cyst originating from a superior labral tear and tracking down the supraspinatus fossa.

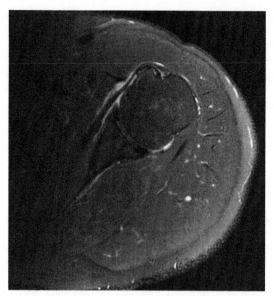

Fig. 5. Axial MR image of a left shoulder shows a tear of the subscapularis with a longitudinal tear within the biceps tendon, with the tendon partially dislocated out of the bicipital groove.

this procedure can be performed using palpable landmarks, ultrasound guidance significantly improves injection accuracy (**Fig. 6**). A randomized clinical trial comparing traditional "landmark" guided injection of the bicipital sheath with ultrasound-guided injection of the bicipital sheath, using contrast dye injection and immediate computed tomography as the gold standard for assessment, found that ultrasound increased injections graded as "only within the tendon sheath" from 26.7% to 86.7%.[35]

NONPHARMACOLOGIC TREATMENT OPTIONS

In addition to anti-inflammatory medications, first-line conservative treatment consists in supervised physiotherapy with a supplemental home exercise program. General

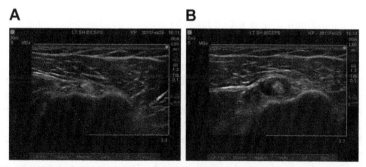

Fig. 6. (*A, B*) Ultrasonographic images in the transverse plane, with the dot in the upper right placed laterally, show an ultrasound-guided injection of the bicipital sheath. (*A*) Preinjection. (*B*) Postinjection. Engorgement of the bicipital sheath with steroid can be seen.

therapy principles apply, such as focusing on range of motion and strengthening of the rotator cuff and periscapular musculature with closed-chain exercises. As malpositioning of the glenoid can worsen symptoms of bicipital tendonitis and SLAP tears, improving scapulothoracic rhythm is critical.[36] Baseball players in particular should focus on stretching of the posterior capsule to restore the rotational arc of the shoulder and counteract the GIRD that commonly develops in these patients.[37] Posterior capsule tightness may contribute to posterosuperior translation of the humeral head, which may place more stress on the labrum and may contribute to the formation, propagation, and symptoms of SLAP tear.[14] Anti-inflammatory modalities such as ice, phonophoresis, and iontophoresis can be used at the discretion of the physical therapist.

SURGICAL TREATMENT OPTIONS

There is no consensus with regard to optimal surgical treatment. Surgical treatment options vary depending on the pathologic status, although the major options include debridement,[38] tenotomy,[39] tenodesis,[1] and, in the case of SLAP tears, SLAP repair.[40] Of note, debridement and SLAP repair preserve the glenohumeral function of the LHBT, whereas tenotomy and tenodesis remove the intra-articular portion of the LHBT and with it any function that this tendon may serve in glenohumeral kinematics.[1]

Glenohumeral Function of the Tendon of the Long Head of the Biceps

The glenohumeral function of the LHBT remains controversial. Whereas some cadaveric studies have suggested that the LHBT may act as a humeral head depressor[41] or a static stabilizer of the glenohumeral joint,[42,43] others have suggested that disruption of the biceps anchor without disrupting the superior labrum may not affect glenohumeral translation.[44] Some in vivo studies have suggested a role for the LHBT as a dynamic stabilizer of the glenohumeral joint,[45] whereas others have demonstrated that the biceps is desynchronized from the remaining glenohumeral musculature, and thus is unlikely to be functionally important.[46] An in vivo biplanar fluoroscopy study demonstrated no alteration of glenohumeral kinematics between biceps tenodesis and normal shoulders.[47] These results are bolstered by several series demonstrating no functional deficits, no instability, no proximal migration, and excellent outcomes in patients status post tenodesis.[39,48]

Arthroscopic Assessment

All operative treatment begins with a full arthroscopic assessment of the biceps and superior labrum. The examiner must be aware of the significant variability in normal anatomy.[20] The anterosuperior labrum may be detached from the glenoid rim with a sublabral foramen, the middle glenohumeral ligament may exist as a cord and insert onto the detached portion, the superior labrum may have a meniscoid appearance, and the biceps may insert onto the superior labrum, the supraglenoid tubercle, or both structures.[20] The examiner must then determine, using a probe, which structures are torn and which have always been anatomically separated. Signs of a SLAP tear include fraying, exposure of glenoid bone, and granulation tissue. In addition, the probe can be used to displace the biceps tendon intra-articularly by manipulating the probe above the tendon and pulling inferiorly. The camera can then be directed anterolaterally down the sheath to visualize the intertubercular portion of the bicipital tendon for erythema, synovitis, or other signs of inflammation, which has been termed the "lipstick lesion" (**Fig. 7**).[20]

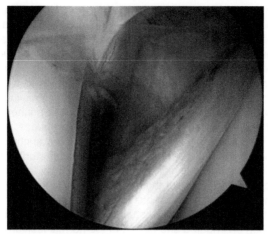

Fig. 7. Arthroscopic image of the right shoulder in the beach-chair position viewed from the posterior portal shows a probe entering from the anterior portal and retracting the biceps intra-articularly. Extensive inflammation and synovitis can be seen on the anterior aspect of the bicipital tendon.

Operative Technique for Repair of Superior Labral Anterior-Posterior Tears

The authors' preference is to perform SLAP repair in the lateral decubitus position. After establishing the posterior portal and performing a diagnostic arthroscopy, 2 portals can be established within the rotator interval, one just off the leading edge of the supraspinatus and the other just above the superior border of the subscapularis. An elevator can be introduced to free any adhesions between the labrum and the glenoid rim. A motorized burr or rasp can be used to prepare the glenoid rim. The authors prefer to retrogradely pass sutures through the chondrolabral junction and capsulolabral junction using a curved, cannulated, suture-passing device (Spectrum; ConMed Linvatec, Largo, FL, USA). Alternating simple and mattress sutures help to recreate the labral bumper in an anatomic position. Knotless anchors (Bioraptor; Smith and Nephew, Andover, MA, USA) are then placed at a dead man's angle at the glenoid articular surface from the most superior portal. In many cases, depending on the patient's anatomy and the tear configuration, transrotator cuff anchor placement will be necessary to achieve the proper position and direction. The authors avoid placing anchors too far anterior to the biceps to avoid overconstraining the anterosuperior capsule, which can contribute to loss of external rotation postoperatively.

Open Subpectoral Biceps Tenodesis

The authors' preference is to perform biceps tenodesis via an open subpectoral approach to avoid potentially leaving residual pathologic biceps tendon within the groove, which can potentially contribute to residual postoperative pain,[49] although comparative studies are undecided as to whether tenodesis site affects outcomes.[50,51] At the completion of the shoulder arthroscopy performed in the beach-chair position, the patient is reclined an additional 20°. Alternatively, in the lateral decubitus position, the patient is rotated back toward a supine position and the arm is outstretched on a Mayo stand to access the subpectoral position. The arm is mildly externally rotated and abducted, and a 3-cm incision is made starting at the inferior edge of the pectoral major insertion within the axilla. After dissection through the subcutaneous tissues, a fascial incision is made between the short head of the biceps medially and the pectoralis major laterally. A retractor can be placed laterally and proximally under the pectoralis and a retractor can be gently placed medially, although the surgeon must exercise care medially because the neurovascular structures, in particular the musculocutaneous nerve,[52] are at risk. The biceps tendon can then be retrieved bluntly from the groove. The authors' preference is to prepare the tendon with a running, stout, reinforced suture at the musculotendinous junction, to remove the remaining proximal tendon and fixate it with an all-suture anchor (Suturefix; Smith and Nephew) at the distal aspect of the groove. Multiple options exist for tenodesis fixation including, among others, an endobutton, a suture anchor, a bone bridge, and a biotenodesis screw. Although some biomechanical studies have suggested the biotenodesis screw to have the highest load to failure in cadaveric specimens,[53,54] no clinical evidence exists to suggest that fixation methodology alters failure rates. In addition, use of an interference screw requires a larger drill hole in the humerus, which may predispose the humerus to spiral fracture,[55] and also incurs additional expense. The wounds can then be irrigated and closed in the normal fashion.

TREATMENT COMPLICATIONS

A wide variety of complications can occur after SLAP repair. Perhaps the most common and difficult to overcome is inability to return to play, which is a multifactorial issue driven by residual pain, inadequate rehabilitation, loss of range of motion, and alterations in proprioception, glenohumeral kinematics, and neuromuscular activation, all of which are difficult to quantify.[56] SLAP repair failure also commonly occurs, likely attributable to the poor vascularity of this region of the labrum.[20] Less commonly encountered complications include arthrofibrosis, chondrolysis, infection, chronic regional pain syndrome, deep venous thromboses, nerve injury either intraoperatively or with the administration or regional anesthesia, and cerebral hypoperfusion in the beach-chair position. In general, acute complications are infrequent: in a recent nationwide database study of shoulder arthroscopies, 30-day complication rates were less than 1%.[57] Complications after subpectoral biceps tenodesis are infrequent. A large series demonstrated a 2% complication rate with open subpectoral tenodesis.[58] One rare complication of particular concern in baseball pitchers is the potential for humeral shaft fracture through the tenodesis site.[59] Other potential complications include infection at the axillary incision, and loss of fixation with cramping and a cosmetic deformity.[58]

EVALUATION OF OUTCOMES
Nonoperative Treatment

Nonoperative treatment, though traditionally suggested as the first line of therapy, may not be successful in all patients. In a recent review of 21 pitchers treated with supervised physical therapy focused on correcting scapular dyskinesia and posterior capsular contracture (GIRD), 40% were able to return to play but only 22% were able to return to their preinjury level of play. However, in this same series those treated surgically also did not do well: return to play was 48% but return to play at the same level was only 7%.[60] Results are much more favorable in lower-level athletes. In another series with mostly recreational athletes, 71% were able to return to preparticipation levels of play, although only 66% of overhead athletes were able to return to the same level of play. However, these investigators did demonstrate significant improvements in pain, function, and quality of life with nonoperative treatment, suggesting that all patients should be treated nonoperatively initially.[61]

Superior Labral Anterior-Posterior Repair

Numerous clinical series have reported outcomes for these procedures.[62,63] Whereas some investigators have reported excellent clinical outcomes with SLAP repair using a variety of clinical outcome measures,[64–66] others have reported more disappointing results, with 40% to 60% patients dissatisfied and experiencing persistent shoulder pain.[67–69] In addition, even in series with good clinical outcomes, the percentage of athletes returning to their preinjury level of play has been unpredictable, with pooled results from a recent systematic review citing a disappointing rate of return to play of 64% (**Table 1**).[62] These results are generally even more disappointing when overhead athletes are isolated (**Table 2**).[63,65,68,70–73] In a recent motion analysis study, pitchers status post SLAP repair were found to have decreased shoulder horizontal abduction, decreased shoulder maximal external rotation, and decreased forward trunk tilt. These alterations may contribute to their difficulty in returning to play.[74]

Biceps Tenodesis

The results of biceps tenodesis for bicipital tendonitis have been consistent and reliable throughout the literature.[1,75,76] In a recent comparative study, both arthroscopic and open subpectoral biceps tenodesis demonstrated excellent American Shoulder and Elbow Surgeons (ASES) scores of 88–90 and Constant scores of 91%–92%.[50] Although biomechanical studies suggest that biceps tenodesis may not restore native joint laxity,[42,43] tenodesis also offers reliable results for patients with failed SLAP repairs. In a recent study of 46 military patients with a minimum 2-year follow-up, ASES scores improved from 68 to 89, and the rate of return to active duty and athletics was 81%.[52]

Comparative Studies

Several studies have been conducted to compare biceps tenodesis and SLAP repair for SLAP tears.[67,77,78] A recent prospective comparative clinical trial in athletes with concomitant rotator cuff repairs comparing SLAP repair with tenodesis, rates of return to preinjury level of play were 37.5% in patients in the repair group versus 100% in the tenodesis group.[67] In the same series, 100% of those patients revised from SLAP

Table 1
Rates of return to play at preinjury levels in past series with SLAP repair

Authors,[Ref] Year	Percentage of Players Returning to Their Previous Level of Play
Fedoriw et al,[60] 2014	7
Boileau et al,[67] 2009	20
Kim et al,[73] 2002	22
O'Brien et al,[79] 2002	52
Ek et al,[77] 2014	60
Enad et al,[80] 2007	62
Yung et al,[70] 2008	69
Brockmeier et al,[64] 2009	74
Ide,[72] 2005	75
Neuman et al,[71] 2011	84
Denard et al,[78] 2014	86
Morgan et al,[66] 1998	87
Paxinos et al,[81] 2006	92

Table 2
Studies comparing outcomes in overhead and nonoverhead athletes with respect to returning to preinjury level of play

Authors,[Ref] Year	Percentage of Players Returning to Their Preinjury Level of Play	
	Overhead Athletes	Nonoverhead Athletes
Kim et al,[73] 2002	22	41
Ide,[72] 2005	60	75
Cohen et al,[68] 2006	37.5	48
Friel et al,[65] 2010	54	NA
Fedoriw et al,[60] 2014	7	NA

Abbreviation: NA, no data available.

repair to tenodesis and 87% of those with primary arthroscopic tenodesis returned their preinjury level of play, although the tenodesis group was older, and this study did not include any overhead-throwing athletes.[67] However, 2 subsequent retrospective studies have failed to show any difference in rates of return to play between biceps tenodesis and SLAP repair, calling these results into question.[77,78] A recent motion analysis study comparing pitchers status post tenodesis with those status post SLAP repair, all of whom were able to return to pitching and were evaluated at least 1 year postoperatively, found altered patterns of thoracic rotation and a suggestion of altered patterns of biceps muscle activation in those who underwent SLAP repair, whereas those who underwent tenodesis more closely resembled normal pitchers.[56]

SUMMARY

The biceps tendon and its anchor at the superior glenoid and labrum is subjected to bicipital tendonitis, instability, and SLAP tears. These disorders are a common cause of pain, particularly in overhead athletes, and specifically among baseball pitchers. However, they can also be encountered in swimmers, tennis players, volleyball players, and softball players. History usually reveals intermittent, activity-related anterolateral shoulder pain worse in "arm-cocking" activities with the shoulder loaded in abducted and external rotation, which causes a dynamic "peel-back" of the posterosuperior labrum. Diagnosis of bicipital tendonitis is driven by tenderness to palpation at the bicipital groove. Diagnosis of SLAP tears is challenging. All patients are initially managed nonoperatively with nonsteroidal anti-inflammatory medications, targeted ultrasound-guided corticosteroid injections, and supervised physical therapy focusing on rotator cuff strengthening, scapular stabilization, and scapular dyskinesis. Options for operative treatment continue to be controversial, and include SLAP repair and biceps tenodesis. Surgical results with biceps tenodesis are consistent and reliable, whereas results with SLAP repair are unpredictable with regard to return to play, especially in overhead athletes and specifically in elite baseball pitchers.

REFERENCES

1. Provencher MT, LeClere LE, Romeo AA. Subpectoral biceps tenodesis. Sports Med Arthrosc 2008;16(3):170–6.
2. Nho SJ, Strauss EJ, Lenart BA, et al. Long head of the biceps tendinopathy: diagnosis and management. J Am Acad Orthop Surg 2010;18(11):645–56.

3. Andrews JR, Carson WG, Mcleod WD. Glenoid labrum tears related to the long head of the biceps. Am J Sports Med 1985;13(5):337–41.

4. Snyder SJ, Banas MP, Karzel RP. An analysis of 140 injuries to the superior glenoid labrum. J Shoulder Elbow Surg 1995;4(4):243–8.

5. Handelberg F, Willems S, Shahabpour M, et al. SLAP lesions: a retrospective multicenter study. Arthroscopy 1998;14(8):856–62.

6. Jain NB, Higgins LD, Losina E, et al. Epidemiology of musculoskeletal upper extremity ambulatory surgery in the United States. BMC Musculoskelet Disord 2014; 15(1):4.

7. Weber S, Martin D, Seiler JI, et al. Incidence rates, complications, and outcomes as reported by the American Board of Orthopaedic Surgery: part II candidates. Am J Sports Med 2012;40(7):1538–43.

8. Werner BC, Brockmeier SF, Gwathmey FW. Trends in long head biceps tenodesis. Am J Sports Med 2014;43(3):570–8.

9. Abrams GD, Safran MR. Diagnosis and management of superior labrum anterior posterior lesions in overhead athletes. Br J Sports Med 2010;44(5):311–8.

10. Fleisig GS, Andrews JR, Dillman CJ, et al. Kinetics of baseball pitching with implications about injury mechanisms. Am J Sports Med 1995;23(2):233–9.

11. Gainor BJ, Piotrowski G, Puhl J, et al. The throw: biomechanics and acute injury. Am J Sports Med 1980;8(2):114–8.

12. Saltzman BM, Chalmers PN, Cornell R, et al. Upper extremity physeal injury in young baseball pitchers. Phys Sportsmed 2014;42(3):100–11.

13. Bey MJ, Elders GJ, Huston LJ, et al. The mechanism of creation of superior labrum, anterior, and posterior lesions in a dynamic biomechanical model of the shoulder: the role of inferior subluxation. J Shoulder Elbow Surg 1998;7(4): 397–401.

14. Burkhart SS, Morgan CD, Kibler WB. Shoulder injuries in overhead athletes. The "dead arm" revisited. Clin Sports Med 2000;19(1):125–58.

15. Burkhart S, Morgan C. SLAP lesions in the overhead athlete. Orthop Clin North Am 2001;32(3):431–41.

16. Burkhart SS, Morgan CD. The peel-back mechanism: its role in producing and extending posterior type II SLAP lesions and its effect on SLAP repair rehabilitation. Arthroscopy 1998;14(6):637–40.

17. Jazrawi L, McCluskey G 3rd, Andrews JR. Superior labral anterior and posterior lesions and internal impingement in the overhead athlete. Instr Course Lect 2003; 52:43–63.

18. Lesniak BP, Baraga MG, Jose J, et al. Glenohumeral findings on magnetic resonance imaging correlate with innings pitched in asymptomatic pitchers. Am J Sports Med 2013;41(9):2022–7.

19. Alpantaki K, McLaughlin D, Karagogeos D, et al. Sympathetic and sensory neural elements in the tendon of the long head of the biceps. J Bone Joint Surg Am 2005;87(7):1580–3.

20. Keener JD, Brophy RH. Superior labral tears of the shoulder: pathogenesis, evaluation, and treatment. J Am Acad Orthop Surg 2009;17(10):627–37.

21. Dines JS, Bedi A, Williams PN, et al. Tennis injuries: epidemiology, pathophysiology, and treatment. J Am Acad Orthop Surg 2015;23(3):181–9.

22. Wu P-T, Jou I-M, Yang C-C, et al. The severity of the long head biceps tendinopathy in patients with chronic rotator cuff tears: macroscopic versus microscopic results. J Shoulder Elbow Surg 2014;23(8):1099–106.

23. Warner J, McMahon PJ. The role of the long head of the biceps brachii in superior stability of the glenohumeral joint. J Bone Joint Surg Am 1995;77(3):366–72.

24. O'Brien SJ, Pagnani MJ, Fealy S, et al. The active compression test: a new and effective test for diagnosing labral tears and acromioclavicular joint abnormality. Am J Sports Med 1998;26(5):610–3.
25. Kim YS, Kim JM, Ha KY, et al. The passive compression test: a new clinical test for superior labral tears of the shoulder. Am J Sports Med 2007;35(9):1489–94.
26. Kibler WB. Specificity and sensitivity of the anterior slide test in throwing athletes with superior glenoid labral tears. Arthroscopy 1995;11(3):296–300.
27. Liu SH, Henry MH, Nuccion SL. A prospective evaluation of a new physical examination in predicting glenoid labral tears. Am J Sports Med 1996;24(6): 721–5.
28. Pandya NK, Colton A, Webner D, et al. Physical examination and magnetic resonance imaging in the diagnosis of superior labrum anterior-posterior lesions of the shoulder: a sensitivity analysis. Arthroscopy 2008;24(3):311–7.
29. Hegedus EJ, Goode A, Campbell S, et al. Physical examination tests of the shoulder: a systematic review with meta-analysis of individual tests. Br J Sports Med 2007;42(2):80–92.
30. Williams MM, Snyder SJ, Buford D. The Buford complex—the "cord-like" middle glenohumeral ligament and absent anterosuperior labrum complex: a normal anatomic capsulolabral variant. Arthroscopy 1994;10(3):241–7.
31. Bhatia S, Chalmers PN, Yanke AB, et al. Arthroscopic suprascapular nerve decompression: transarticular and subacromial approach. Arthrosc Tech 2012; 1(2):e187–92.
32. Sheridan K, Kreulen C, Kim S, et al. Accuracy of magnetic resonance imaging to diagnose superior labrum anterior-posterior tears. Knee Surg Sports Traumatol Arthrosc 2015;23(9):2645–50.
33. Schaeffeler C, Waldt S, Holzapfel K, et al. Lesions of the biceps pulley: diagnostic accuracy of MR arthrography of the shoulder and evaluation of previously described and new diagnostic signs. Radiology 2012;264(2):504–13.
34. Yablon CM, Bedi A, Morag Y, et al. Ultrasonography of the shoulder with arthroscopic correlation. Clin Sports Med 2013;32(3):391–408.
35. Hashiuchi T, Sakurai G, Morimoto M, et al. Accuracy of the biceps tendon sheath injection: ultrasound-guided or unguided injection? A randomized controlled trial. J Shoulder Elbow Surg 2011;20(7):1069–73.
36. Kibler WB. The role of the scapula in athletic shoulder function. Am J Sports Med 1998;26(2):325–37.
37. Wilk KE, Macrina LC, Fleisig GS, et al. Deficits in glenohumeral passive range of motion increase risk of elbow injury in professional baseball pitchers: a prospective study. Am J Sports Med 2014;42(9):2075–81.
38. Cordasco FA, Steinmann S, Flatow EL, et al. Arthroscopic treatment of glenoid labral tears. Am J Sports Med 1993;21(3):425–30 [discussion: 430–1].
39. Boileau P, Baque F, Valerio L, et al. Isolated arthroscopic biceps tenotomy or tenodesis improves symptoms in patients with massive irreparable rotator cuff tears. J Bone Joint Surg Am 2007;89(4):747–57.
40. Frank RM, Nho SJ, McGill KC, et al. Retrospective analysis of arthroscopic superior labrum anterior to posterior repair: prognostic factors associated with failure. Adv Orthop 2013;2013(8):1–7.
41. Kumar VP, Satku K, Balasubramaniam P. The role of the long head of biceps brachii in the stabilization of the head of the humerus. Clin Orthop Relat Res 1989; 244:172–5.
42. Strauss EJ, Salata MJ, Sershon RA, et al. Role of the superior labrum after biceps tenodesis in glenohumeral stability. J Shoulder Elbow Surg 2014;23(4):485–91.

43. Patzer T, Habermeyer P, Hurschler C, et al. The influence of superior labrum anterior to posterior (SLAP) repair on restoring baseline glenohumeral translation and increased biceps loading after simulated SLAP tear and the effectiveness of SLAP repair after long head of biceps tenotomy. J Shoulder Elbow Surg 2012; 21(11):1580–7.

44. Pagnani MJ, Deng XH, Warren RF, et al. Effect of lesions of the superior portion of the glenoid labrum on glenohumeral translation. J Bone Joint Surg Am 1995; 77(7):1003–10.

45. Chalmers PN, Cip J, Trombley R, et al. Glenohumeral function of the long head of the biceps muscle: an electromyographic analysis. Orthop J Sports Med 2014; 2(2). http://dx.doi.org/10.1177/2325967114523902.

46. Hawkes DH, Alizadehkhaiyat O, Fisher AC, et al. Normal shoulder muscular activation and co-ordination during a shoulder elevation task based on activities of daily living: an electromyographic study. J Orthop Res 2011;30(1):53–60.

47. Giphart JE, Elser F, Dewing CB, et al. The long head of the biceps tendon has minimal effect on in vivo glenohumeral kinematics: a biplane fluoroscopy study. Am J Sports Med 2012;40(1):202–12.

48. Boileau P, Krishnan SG, Coste J-S, et al. Arthroscopic biceps tenodesis: a new technique using bioabsorbable interference screw fixation. Arthroscopy 2002; 18(9):1002–12.

49. Moon SC, Cho NS, Rhee YG. Analysis of "hidden lesions" of the extra-articular biceps after subpectoral biceps tenodesis: the subpectoral portion as the optimal tenodesis site. Am J Sports Med 2015;43(1):63–8.

50. Werner BC, Evans CL, Holzgrefe RE, et al. Arthroscopic suprapectoral and open subpectoral biceps tenodesis: a comparison of minimum 2-year clinical outcomes. Am J Sports Med 2014;42(11):2583–90.

51. Lutton DM, Gruson KI, Harrison AK, et al. Where to tenodese the biceps: proximal or distal? Clin Orthop Relat Res 2011;469(4):1050–5.

52. McCormick F, Nwachukwu B, Solomon D, et al. The efficacy of biceps tenodesis in the treatment of failed superior labral anterior posterior repairs. Am J Sports Med 2014;42(4):820–5.

53. Golish SR, Caldwell PE III, Miller MD, et al. Interference screw versus suture anchor fixation for subpectoral tenodesis of the proximal biceps tendon: a cadaveric study. Arthroscopy 2008;24(10):1103–8.

54. Mazzocca AD, Bicos J, Santangelo S, et al. The biomechanical evaluation of four fixation techniques for proximal biceps tenodesis. Arthroscopy 2005;21(11): 1296–306.

55. Reiff SN, Nho SJ, Romeo AA. Proximal humerus fracture after keyhole biceps tenodesis. Am J Orthop 2010;39(7):E61–3.

56. Chalmers PN, Trombley R, Cip J, et al. Postoperative restoration of upper extremity motion and neuromuscular control during the overhand pitch: evaluation of tenodesis and repair for superior labral anterior-posterior tears. Am J Sports Med 2014;42(12):2825–36.

57. Martin CT, Gao Y, Pugely AJ, et al. 30-day morbidity and mortality after elective shoulder arthroscopy: a review of 9410 cases. J Shoulder Elbow Surg 2013; 22(12):1667–75.e1.

58. Nho SJ, Reiff SN, Verma NN, et al. Complications associated with subpectoral biceps tenodesis: low rates of incidence following surgery. J Shoulder Elbow Surg 2010;19(5):764–8.

59. Heckman DS, Creighton RA, Romeo AA. Management of failed biceps tenodesis or tenotomy: causation and treatment. Sports Med Arthrosc 2010;18(3):173–80.

60. Fedoriw WW, Ramkumar P, McCulloch PC, et al. Return to play after treatment of superior labral tears in professional baseball players. Am J Sports Med 2014; 42(5):1155–60.

61. Edwards SL, Lee JA, Bell J-E, et al. Nonoperative treatment of superior labrum anterior posterior tears: improvements in pain, function, and quality of life. Am J Sports Med 2010;38(7):1456–61.

62. Gorantla K, Gill C, Wright RW. The outcome of type II SLAP repair: a systematic review. Arthroscopy 2010;26(4):537–45.

63. Sayde WM, Cohen SB, Ciccotti MG, et al. Return to play after Type II superior labral anterior-posterior lesion repairs in athletes: a systematic review. Clin Orthop Relat Res 2012;470(6):1595–600.

64. Brockmeier SF, Voos JE, Williams RJ, et al. Outcomes after arthroscopic repair of type-II SLAP lesions. J Bone Joint Surg Am 2009;91(7):1595–603.

65. Friel NA, Karas V, Slabaugh MA, et al. Outcomes of type II superior labrum, anterior to posterior (SLAP) repair: Prospective evaluation at a minimum two-year follow-up. J Shoulder Elbow Surg 2010;19(6):859–67.

66. Morgan CD, Burkhart SS, Palmeri M, et al. Type II SLAP lesions: three subtypes and their relationships to superior instability and rotator cuff tears. Arthroscopy 1998;14(6):553–65.

67. Boileau P, Parratte S, Chuinard C, et al. Arthroscopic treatment of isolated type II SLAP lesions: biceps tenodesis as an alternative to reinsertion. Am J Sports Med 2009;37(5):929–36.

68. Cohen DB, Coleman S, Drakos MC, et al. Outcomes of isolated type II SLAP lesions treated with arthroscopic fixation using a bioabsorbable tack. Arthroscopy 2006;22(2):136–42.

69. Verma NN, Garretson R, Romeo AA. Outcome of arthroscopic repair of type II SLAP lesions in worker's compensation patients. HSS J 2006;3(1):58–62.

70. Yung PS-H, Fong DT-P, Kong M-F, et al. Arthroscopic repair of isolated type II superior labrum anterior-posterior lesion. Knee Surg Sports Traumatol Arthrosc 2008;16(12):1151–7.

71. Neuman BJ, Boisvert CB, Reiter B, et al. Results of arthroscopic repair of type II superior labral anterior posterior lesions in overhead athletes: assessment of return to preinjury playing level and satisfaction. Am J Sports Med 2011;39(9): 1883–8.

72. Ide J. Sports activity after arthroscopic superior labral repair using suture anchors in overhead-throwing athletes. Am J Sports Med 2005;33(4):507–14.

73. Kim S-H, Ha K-I, Kim S-H, et al. Results of arthroscopic treatment of superior labral lesions. J Bone Joint Surg Am 2002;84-A(6):981–5.

74. Laughlin WA, Fleisig GS, Scillia AJ, et al. Deficiencies in pitching biomechanics in baseball players with a history of superior labrum anterior-posterior repair. Am J Sports Med 2014;42(12):2837–41.

75. Mazzocca AD, Rios CG, Romeo AA, et al. Subpectoral biceps tenodesis with interference screw fixation. Arthroscopy 2005;21(7):896.e1–7.

76. Romeo AA, Mazzocca AD, Tauro JC. Arthroscopic biceps tenodesis. Arthroscopy 2004;20(2):206–13.

77. Ek ETH, Shi LL, Tompson JD, et al. Surgical treatment of isolated type II superior labrum anterior-posterior (SLAP) lesions: repair versus biceps tenodesis. J Shoulder Elbow Surg 2014;23(7):1059–65.

78. Denard PJ, Lädermann A, Parsley BK, et al. Arthroscopic biceps tenodesis compared with repair of isolated type II SLAP lesions in patients older than 35 years. Orthopedics 2014;37(3):e292–7.

79. O'Brien SJ, Allen AA, Coleman SH, et al. The trans-rotator cuff approach to SLAP lesions: technical aspects for repair and a clinical follow-up of 31 patients at a minimum of 2 years. Arthroscopy 2002;18(4):372–7.

80. Enad JG, Gaines RJ, White SM, et al. Arthroscopic superior labrum anterior-posterior repair in military patients. J Shoulder Elbow Surg 2007;16(3):300–5.

81. Paxinos A, Walton J, Rütten S, et al. Arthroscopic stabilization of superior labral (SLAP) tears with biodegradable tack: outcomes to 2 years. Arthroscopy 2006; 22(6):627–34.

Complications of Proximal Biceps Tenotomy and Tenodesis

Mandeep S. Virk, MD[a,b], Gregory P. Nicholson, MD[a,b,*]

KEYWORDS

- Biceps tenotomy • Biceps tenodesis • Complication

KEY POINTS

- Tenotomy of the LHBT tendon is a safe and quick procedure but can result in cosmetic deformity and cramping or soreness in the biceps muscle.
- Tenodesis of the LHBT provides a new, distal level of fixation for the tenotomized tendon and results in lower risk of cosmetic deformity or cramping in the biceps muscle.
- Tenodesis of the LHBT has an overall low complication rate but complications can be severe and include neurologic injuries, proximal humerus fracture, reflex sympathetic dystrophy, and infection.

INTRODUCTION

The long head of the biceps tendon (LHBT) has a unique anatomy, but with a less understood functional role in glenohumeral joint stability.[1] The proximal part of the LHBT is relatively fixed at its origin on the supraglenoid tubercle and the superior labrum. After a brief intra-articular course where it is mobile, the tendon makes a sharp turn into the bicipital groove. Within the bicipital groove, the tendon is again relatively anchored. This relative fixation of the proximal part of the LHBT at two sites in the setting of extensive mobility of the glenohumeral joint predisposes the LHBT to high stresses. The LHBT can be affected by inflammation, trauma, impingement, instability (typically associated with subscapularis tears), intrinsic degeneration, and fibrosis in the rotator interval.[2,3]

The functional significance of the LHBT remains a topic of debate, but the LHBT is a recognized source of anterior shoulder pain.[3] Pathologic involvement of the LHBT is

a Division of Shoulder and Elbow, Department of Orthopaedic Surgery, Rush University Medical Center, 1611 West Harrison Street, Chicago, IL 60612, USA; b Division of Sports Medicine, Department of Orthopaedic Surgery, Rush University Medical Center, 1611 West Harrison Street, Chicago, IL 60612, USA
* Corresponding author. Division of Sports Medicine, Department of Orthopaedic Surgery, Rush University Medical Center, 1611 West Harrison Street, Chicago, IL 60612.
E-mail address: gregory.nicholson@rushortho.com

Clin Sports Med 35 (2016) 181–188
http://dx.doi.org/10.1016/j.csm.2015.08.011   sportsmed.theclinics.com
0278-5919/16/$ – see front matter © 2016 Elsevier Inc. All rights reserved.

usually seen in association with rotator cuff tears, shoulder arthritis, shoulder trauma, and labral pathology, which makes it challenging to determine the contribution or role of the LHBT in shoulder pain. The clinical tests for the LHBT pathology are neither sensitive nor specific.[4]

Tenotomy and tenodesis of the LHBT are two surgical treatment options for addressing the LHBT pathology.[5–10] Tenotomy of the LHBT relieves pain by preventing traction insult to the inflamed, torn, or degenerated biceps tendon. Proponents of the biceps tenotomy believe that it is a simple and safe procedure that consistently relieves pain and allows quicker rehabilitation compared with biceps tenodesis.[11,12] In contrast, tenodesis eliminates proximal tendon angulation, provides a new fixation anchor for the tenotomized tendon in the proximal humerus, and thus maintains the length-tension relationship of the LHBT musculotendinous unit.[13,14] However, the tenodesis site has to be protected and requires an initial period of immobilization. Biceps tenotomy and tenodesis are associated with specific limitations and complications, which can affect the clinical outcome and influence patient satisfaction postoperatively.

COMPLICATIONS OF BICEPS TENOTOMY

Multiple studies have reported a high satisfaction rate after biceps tenotomy.[5,11,12,15,16] Cosmetic deformity of the arm, cramping or soreness in the biceps muscle, and strength deficits in elbow flexion and supination are the three most commonly reported adverse events associated with the biceps tenotomy.[5,11,12,16] Tenotomizing the LHBT results in variable degrees of distal migration of the biceps tendon, which can result in cosmetic deformity including the "Popeye" sign (**Fig. 1**). The severity of cosmetic deformity after biceps tenotomy varies and patient perception of the deformity is also variable. Elderly patients are less affected by the cosmetic outcome compared with younger patients.[11,12] Cramping, soreness, or fatigue sensation in the biceps muscle can also occur after biceps tenotomy and is probably related to loss of proximal anchorage of the LHBT. However, not every biceps tenotomy is associated with a Popeye sign or biceps cramping and prevalence of these complications is variable in the reported literature.[5,11,12,15,16] Biceps tenotomy can result in perception of weakness of elbow strength. Objective strength measurement studies have demonstrated loss of elbow flexion and supination strength in the operative arm compared with the contralateral arm or nonoperative control arms.[17,18] However, the weakness in elbow strength after biceps tenotomy is more of a concern in the

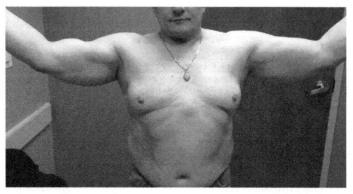

Fig. 1. Posttenotomy Popeye deformity in the arm.

young, active patient, such as a manual laborer, and is often inconsequential in older, sedentary patients.

Gill and colleagues[15] reported a complication rate of approximately 13% in a retrospective cohort analysis of arthroscopic biceps tenotomy in 30 patients. Preoperative diagnosis in the cohort group included biceps tendinitis with or without impingement, partial tear of the LHBT, type IV SLAP lesion, anterior instability, and supraspinatus tear. Four patients had poor results after biceps tenotomy. One patient complained of cosmetic deformity and underwent biceps tenodesis, one patient continued to complain of persistent pain, and two other patients had loss of overhead function secondary to impingement syndrome. Kelly and colleagues[12] reported a Popeye sign in 70% of the patients (N = 40) that underwent arthroscopic biceps tenotomy for isolated LHBT tendinitis or LHBT involvement in the presence of concomitant pathology (rotator cuff tears, degenerative joint disease, impingement, shoulder instability, or adhesive capsulitis). There were clinically significant strength deficits in the operative arm compared with the contralateral arm in young patients but not in those age 60 years or greater. Thirty-two percent of people self-rated their outcome as fair or poor. All the patients with poor results had concomitant procedures performed (rotator cuff repair, joint debridement, and acromioplasty). Fatigue discomfort isolated to the biceps muscle after resisted elbow flexion was present in 37.5% of the patients. Interestingly, patients who were more than 60 years old did not have this complication.

In a retrospective cohort analysis of 117 patients that underwent biceps tenotomy, Duff and Campbell[11] reported a satisfaction rate of 95%. Twenty-seven percent of the patients noticed a cosmetic deformity and 19% patients had cramping sensation in the biceps. Thirty-one percent of patients reported weakness in their operative extremity, although there was no significant difference in the objective testing of elbow flexion and supination strength compared with the contralateral arm. In a large cohort of 307 patients that underwent arthroscopic biceps tenotomy as a part of the treatment of irreparable rotator cuff tears, Walch and colleagues[16] reported an 87% satisfaction rate after this procedure. Approximately 50% of the patients noticed a cosmetic deformity. There were no complaints of weakness in elbow flexion or supination. However, no objective strength testing was performed. In a retrospective study of 39 patients that underwent arthroscopic biceps tenotomy for the treatment of irreparable rotator cuff tears, Boileau and colleagues[5] reported a 72% satisfaction rate with the procedure. A Popeye sign was present in 62% of the shoulders. However, only 16 patients noticed the deformity and no patient was bothered by the cosmetic deformity. Twenty-one percent of the patients reported muscular cramping and 46% reported pain in the bicipital groove.

The previously mentioned retrospective case series and case control studies demonstrate that biceps tenotomy is an effective treatment option in a select patient population and has a low revision rate. The incidence of biceps cramping, loss of elbow flexion and supination strength, and concerns regarding cosmetic deformity are relatively less pronounced in the elderly patient population and seldom require revision surgery. However, cosmetic concerns can be important in young, thinner patients and loss of elbow strength, especially supination strength, may result in poor satisfaction in manual laborers.

COMPLICATIONS OF BICEPS TENODESIS

Biceps tenodesis provides a new fixation point for the tenotomized LHBT and thus maintains the length-tension relationship of the LHBT musculotendinous unit.[14,19,20] Compared with biceps tenotomy, the advantages of tenodesis include a lower risk of postoperative cramping or loss of elbow flexion and supination strength and improved cosmetic results. However, biceps tenodesis is a more complex operation that requires a period of postoperative immobilization and lengthier rehabilitation. There are numerous techniques and implants available for the tenodesis of the LHBT. Bone tunnels and key-hole techniques tenodese the tendon to the bone but do not require the use of implants.[21,22] Similarly, soft tissue tenodesis to the conjoint tendon, pectoralis major, or rotator cuff does not require any special implant for fixation.[23] Alternately, the LHBT can be tenodesed to bone using an interference screw, an endobutton, or a suture anchor.[24–26] Although considered a safe procedure, biceps tenodesis is associated with complications that are different than biceps tenotomy. The complications from biceps tenodesis are categorized into the following complications common to all types of tenodesis, and complications related to tenodesis technique (open vs arthroscopic; soft tissue vs bony tenodesis) or implant-specific complications.

Complications common to all types of tenodesis
a. Length-tension mismatch
b. Loss of fixation and occurrence of deformity
c. Biceps pain
d. Shoulder stiffness
e. Infection
 f. Hematoma
g. Neurologic injuries
h. Vascular injuries
 i. Reflex sympathetic dystrophy

Tenodesis technique or implant-specific complications
a. Proximal groove pain
b. Proximal humerus fracture
c. Implant failure
d. Bioabsorbable screw reaction

There is debate regarding the optimal anatomic location for tenodesis, ideal implant for tenodesis, and open versus arthroscopic techniques for tenodesis.[6,9,27–30] The LHBT tenodesis can be performed at a suprapectoral or subpectoral location. There is no consensus on the optimal level of tenodesis in the proximal humerus.[28,29,31,32] Furthermore, there is no high-quality evidence to recommend one surgical technique over the other. The proponents of distal, subpectoral fixation believe that removal of the LHBT and tenosynovium from the bicipital groove allows the surgeon to avoid residual "groove pain," which is believed to originate from the intertubercular part of the LHBT that may be scarred or inflamed. Retrospective case studies by Lutton and colleagues[28] and Sanders and colleagues[32] have reported a higher complication rate and residual groove pain with proximal, suprapectoral biceps tenodesis. However, in a recently reported large series of arthroscopic proximal biceps tenodesis (1083 cases), Brady and colleagues[13] reported a biceps tenodesis–specific complication rate of 0.4%, which included three symptomatic ruptures and one patient with biceps pain. All patients had an arthroscopic proximal biceps tenodesis using an interference screw at the most proximal part of the biceps groove but no patient had proximal biceps groove pain.[13] Gombera and colleagues[31] compared 23 patients that underwent arthroscopic suprapectoral tenodesis with 23 patients that underwent open subpectoral biceps tenodesis and found no significant difference in the pain relief or occurrence of Popeye deformity.

Proximal humerus fracture is a rare but recognized complication associated with tenodesis techniques that involve drilling bigger cortical tunnels (key hole, interference screw fixation), which can serve as a stress riser in the proximal humeral shaft.[33–36] The fractures present within the first few months after surgery, and are oblique or spiral shaped in pattern. Sears and colleagues[33] reported two cases of proximal humerus shaft fracture in young, healthy subjects within 1 year after subpectoral biceps tenodesis with an interference screw fixation. Both patients required open reduction and internal fixation for management of their fractures. Proximal humerus fracture after open subpectoral biceps tenodesis or key-hole tenodesis has been reported by Dein and colleagues,[34] Reiff and colleagues,[35] and Friedel and colleagues[36] as single patient case reports.

Complications common to all types of biceps tenodesis procedure include loss of fixation, infection, hematoma, neurologic injuries, vascular injuries, and reflex sympathetic dystrophy.[19,20,37] The incidence of these complications has been reported to be very low (<1%). Although not frequently reported, the authors believe that LHBT length-tension mismatch can result in a poor patient satisfaction after biceps tenodesis. Loss of fixation and biceps pain are the most commonly reported complication after biceps tenodesis. The failure of fixation can occur at the implant-bone interface or the implant-tendon interface.[37,38] In our experience, the implant-tendon interface failure is more common. Although cadaveric biomechanical studies comparing different fixation methods demonstrate that interference screw fixation offers maximum pullout strength, no clinical studies have compared failure rates with different tenodesis devices.[39] It has been suggested that loss of fixation with occurrence of a Popeye deformity occurs more commonly than previously thought, although not all patients are bothered by it.[24] Biceps cramping and pain at the tenodesis site can occur but the incidence is low compared with the tenotomy. In a consecutive series of 84 arthroscopic biceps tenodesis using a suture anchor in the bicipital groove, Lee and colleagues[24] reported a 25% incidence of MRI-proved distal migration of the LHBT. Interestingly, only 11 patients (12.9%) were diagnosed with the deformity and only two patients noticed the deformity. Mazzocca and colleagues[39] studied 41 patients at approximately 1 year after open subpectoral biceps tenodesis. There was one fixation failure caused by rerupture of the tendon (2%). Nho and colleagues[37] reported the incidence of complications following open subpectoral biceps tenodesis in a cohort of 353 patients over a 3-year period. The overall complication rate was 2%. Complications included persistent bicipital pain (0.57%), failure of fixation (0.57%), infection (0.28%), musculocutaneous neuropathy (0.28%), and reflex sympathetic dystrophy (0.28%).

Neurovascular complications are rare but are seen more commonly with the open biceps tenodesis techniques.[37,40] Anatomic cadaveric experiments have studied the relationship and proximity of various neurovascular structures including the musculocutaneous, radial, median, ulnar, and axillary nerves and brachial artery to the biceps tenodesis site.[41,42] The relationship of neurovascular structures to the bicipital groove gets distorted with arm swelling secondary to arthroscopic fluid leaking in the subacromial and subdeltoid spaces during shoulder arthroscopy. This is especially true when biceps tenodesis is performed in conjunction with rotator cuff repair or labral repair because it is usually the final part of the procedure. The musculocutaneous nerve is the most commonly reported nerve injury in biceps tenodesis, especially with open subpectoral biceps tenodesis. Rhee and colleagues[43] reported four cases of brachial plexus injury in association with open subpectoral biceps tenodesis. Nho and colleagues[37] reported one case of musculocutaneous neuropathy in their series of 353 patients that underwent open subpectoral biceps tenodesis with an

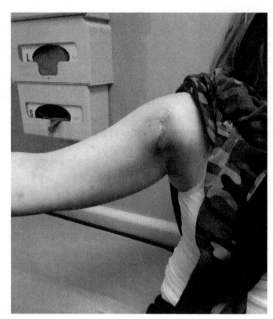

Fig. 2. Deep infection after open biceps tenodesis.

interference screw. The authors recommend careful use of medial retractors and thorough identification of the LHBT before the retrieving the tendon and performing the tenodesis procedure.

Infection (**Fig. 2**), rupture at the LHBT musculotendinous junction when retrieving the tendon out of the groove, adverse reaction to the implant, and reflex sympathetic dystrophy are rare but reported complications in the literature.

SUMMARY

The LHBT is a recognized cause of anterior shoulder pain. Tenotomy and tenodesis of the LHBT are effective in relieving pain arising from the LHBT. Tenotomy is a quick and safe surgery but is limited by a high rate of postoperative cosmetic deformity, and cramping or soreness in the biceps muscle. Tenodesis of LHBT, however, has a lower risk of cosmetic deformity and cramping in the biceps muscle, but can result in more severe complications, such as neurologic injuries, proximal humerus fracture, reflex sympathetic dystrophy, and infection. Fortunately, these serious complications are uncommon and are minimized by improved understanding of regional anatomy, especially the medial neurovascular bundle, and careful placement of medial retractors in open tenodesis techniques.

REFERENCES

1. Hussain WM, Reddy D, Atanda A, et al. The longitudinal anatomy of the long head of the biceps tendon and implications on tenodesis. Knee Surg Sports Traumatol Arthrosc 2015;23:1518–23.
2. Murthi AM, Vosburgh CL, Neviaser TJ. The incidence of pathologic changes of the long head of the biceps tendon. J Shoulder Elbow Surg 2000;9:382–5.

3. Szabo I, Boileau P, Walch G. The proximal biceps as a pain generator and results of tenotomy. Sports Med Arthrosc 2008;16:180–6.
4. Ben Kibler W, Sciascia AD, Hester P, et al. Clinical utility of traditional and new tests in the diagnosis of biceps tendon injuries and superior labrum anterior and posterior lesions in the shoulder. Am J Sports Med 2009;37:1840–7.
5. Boileau P, Baque F, Valerio L, et al. Isolated arthroscopic biceps tenotomy or tenodesis improves symptoms in patients with massive irreparable rotator cuff tears. J Bone Jointt Surg Am 2007;89:747–57.
6. Delle Rose G, Borroni M, Silvestro A, et al. The long head of biceps as a source of pain in active population: tenotomy or tenodesis? A comparison of 2 case series with isolated lesions. Musculoskelet Surg 2012;96(Suppl 1):S47–52.
7. Frost A, Zafar MS, Maffulli N. Tenotomy versus tenodesis in the management of pathologic lesions of the tendon of the long head of the biceps brachii. Am J Sports Med 2009;37:828–33.
8. Hsu AR, Ghodadra NS, Provencher MT, et al. Biceps tenotomy versus tenodesis: a review of clinical outcomes and biomechanical results. J Shoulder Elbow Surg 2011;20:326–32.
9. Koh KH, Ahn JH, Kim SM, et al. Treatment of biceps tendon lesions in the setting of rotator cuff tears: prospective cohort study of tenotomy versus tenodesis. Am J Sports Med 2010;38:1584–90.
10. Slenker NR, Lawson K, Ciccotti MG, et al. Biceps tenotomy versus tenodesis: clinical outcomes. Arthroscopy 2012;28:576–82.
11. Duff SJ, Campbell PT. Patient acceptance of long head of biceps brachii tenotomy. J Shoulder Elbow Surg 2012;21:61–5.
12. Kelly AM, Drakos MC, Fealy S, et al. Arthroscopic release of the long head of the biceps tendon: functional outcome and clinical results. Am J Sports Med 2005; 33:208–13.
13. Brady PC, Narbona P, Adams CR, et al. Arthroscopic proximal biceps tenodesis at the articular margin: evaluation of outcomes, complications, and revision rate. Arthroscopy 2015;31:470–6.
14. Mazzocca AD, Rios CG, Romeo AA, et al. Subpectoral biceps tenodesis with interference screw fixation. Arthroscopy 2005;21:896.
15. Gill TJ, McIrvin E, Mair SD, et al. Results of biceps tenotomy for treatment of pathology of the long head of the biceps brachii. J Shoulder Elbow Surg 2001;10:247–9.
16. Walch G, Edwards TB, Boulahia A, et al. Arthroscopic tenotomy of the long head of the biceps in the treatment of rotator cuff tears: clinical and radiographic results of 307 cases. J Shoulder Elbow Surg 2005;14:238–46.
17. Shank JR, Singleton SB, Braun S, et al. A comparison of forearm supination and elbow flexion strength in patients with long head of the biceps tenotomy or tenodesis. Arthroscopy 2011;27:9–16.
18. Wittstein JR, Queen R, Abbey A, et al. Isokinetic strength, endurance, and subjective outcomes after biceps tenotomy versus tenodesis: a postoperative study. Am J Sports Med 2011;39:857–65.
19. Nho SJ, Strauss EJ, Lenart BA, et al. Long head of the biceps tendinopathy: diagnosis and management. J Am Acad Orthop Surg 2010;18:645–56.
20. Werner BC, Brockmeier SF, Gwathmey FW. Trends in long head biceps tenodesis. Am J Sports Med 2015;43:570–8.
21. Said HG, Babaqi AA, Mohamadean A, et al. Modified subpectoral biceps tenodesis. Int Orthop 2014;38:1063–6.
22. Froimson AI, O I. Keyhole tenodesis of biceps origin at the shoulder. Clin Orthop Relat Res 1975;(112):245–9.

23. Drakos MC, Verma NN, Gulotta LV, et al. Arthroscopic transfer of the long head of the biceps tendon: functional outcome and clinical results. Arthroscopy 2008;24: 217–23.

24. Lee HI, Shon MS, Koh KH, et al. Clinical and radiologic results of arthroscopic biceps tenodesis with suture anchor in the setting of rotator cuff tear. J Shoulder Elbow Surg 2014;23:e53–60.

25. Mazzocca AD, Cote MP, Arciero CL, et al. Clinical outcomes after subpectoral biceps tenodesis with an interference screw. Am J Sports Med 2008;36:1922–9.

26. Snir N, Hamula M, Wolfson T, et al. Long head of the biceps tenodesis with cortical button technique. Arthrosc Tech 2013;2:e95–7.

27. Friedman DJ, Dunn JC, Higgins LD, et al. Proximal biceps tendon: injuries and management. Sports Med Arthrosc 2008;16:162–9.

28. Lutton DM, Gruson KI, Harrison AK, et al. Where to tenodese the biceps: proximal or distal? Clin Orthop Relat Res 2011;469:1050–5.

29. Werner BC, Evans CL, Holzgrefe RE, et al. Arthroscopic suprapectoral and open subpectoral biceps tenodesis: a comparison of minimum 2-year clinical outcomes. Am J Sports Med 2014;42:2583–90.

30. Osbahr DC, Diamond AB, Speer KP. The cosmetic appearance of the biceps muscle after long-head tenotomy versus tenodesis. Arthroscopy 2002;18:483–7.

31. Gombera MM, Kahlenberg CA, Nair R, et al. All-arthroscopic suprapectoral versus open subpectoral tenodesis of the long head of the biceps brachii. Am J Sports Med 2015;43:1077–83.

32. Sanders B, Lavery KP, Pennington S, et al. Clinical success of biceps tenodesis with and without release of the transverse humeral ligament. J Shoulder Elbow Surg 2012;21:66–71.

33. Sears BW, Spencer EE, Getz CL. Humeral fracture following subpectoral biceps tenodesis in 2 active, healthy patients. J Shoulder Elbow Surg 2011;20:e7–11.

34. Dein EJ, Huri G, Gordon JC, et al. A humerus fracture in a baseball pitcher after biceps tenodesis. Am J Sports Med 2014;42:877–9.

35. Reiff SN, Nho SJ, Romeo AA. Proximal humerus fracture after keyhole biceps tenodesis. Am J Orthop 2010;39:E61–3.

36. Friedel R, Markgraf E, Schmidt I, et al. Proximal humerus shaft fracture as a complication after keyhole-plasty. A case report. Unfallchirurgie 1995;21: 198–201 [in German].

37. Nho SJ, Reiff SN, Verma NN, et al. Complications associated with subpectoral biceps tenodesis: low rates of incidence following surgery. J Shoulder Elbow Surg 2010;19:764–8.

38. Koch BS, Burks RT. Failure of biceps tenodesis with interference screw fixation. Arthroscopy 2012;28:735–40.

39. Mazzocca AD, Bicos J, Santangelo S, et al. The biomechanical evaluation of four fixation techniques for proximal biceps tenodesis. Arthroscopy 2005;21:1296–306.

40. Ma H, Van Heest A, Glisson C, et al. Musculocutaneous nerve entrapment: an unusual complication after biceps tenodesis. Am J Sports Med 2009;37:2467–9.

41. Dickens JF, Kilcoyne KG, Tintle SM, et al. Subpectoral biceps tenodesis: an anatomic study and evaluation of at-risk structures. Am J Sports Med 2012;40: 2337–41.

42. Ding DY, Gupta A, Snir N, et al. Nerve proximity during bicortical drilling for subpectoral biceps tenodesis: a cadaveric study. Arthroscopy 2014;30:942–6.

43. Rhee PC, Spinner RJ, Bishop AT, et al. Iatrogenic brachial plexus injuries associated with open subpectoral biceps tenodesis: a report of 4 cases. Am J Sports Med 2013;41:2048–53.

Index

Note: Page numbers of article titles are in **boldface** type.

Clin Sports Med 35 (2016) 189–193
http://dx.doi.org/10.1016/S0278-5919(15)00120-9
0278-5919/16/$ – see front matter © 2016 Elsevier Inc. All rights reserved.

Moving?

Make sure your subscription moves with you!

To notify us of your new address, find your **Clinics Account Number** (located on your mailing label above your name), and contact customer service at:

Email: journalscustomerservice-usa@elsevier.com

800-654-2452 (subscribers in the U.S. & Canada)
314-447-8871 (subscribers outside of the U.S. & Canada)

Fax number: 314-447-8029

Elsevier Health Sciences Division
Subscription Customer Service
3251 Riverport Lane
Maryland Heights, MO 63043

*To ensure uninterrupted delivery of your subscription, please notify us at least 4 weeks in advance of move.